Team Nutrition's

Food, Family and Fun

A Seasonal Guide to Healthy Eating

Commemorating 50 years of School Lunch

USDA's TEAM NUTRITION

Mission

To improve the health and education of children by creating innovative public and private partnerships that promote food choices for a healthful diet through the media, schools, families, and the community.

Principles

Supporters of Team Nutrition share these common values:

1. We believe that children should be empowered to make food choices that reflect the Dietary Guidelines for Americans.
2. We believe that good nutrition and physical activity are essential to children's health and educational success.
3. We believe that school meals that meet the Dietary Guidelines for Americans should appeal to children and taste good.
4. We believe our programs must build upon the best science, education, communication and technical resources available.
5. We believe that public/private partnerships are essential to reaching children to promote food choices for a healthful diet.
6. We believe that messages to children should be age appropriate and delivered in a language they speak, through media they use, in ways that are entertaining and actively involve them in learning.
7. We believe in focusing on positive messages regarding food choices children can make.
8. We believe it is critical to stimulate and support action and education at the national, state and local levels to successfully change children's eating behaviors.

Acknowledgments

We want to thank the nearly 40 volunteer chefs, credited in the seasonal recipe sections, and other Team Nutrition supporters around the country who made this book possible. For their enthusiasm, ideas, numerous conference calls, suggestions, and recipes, we are very grateful.

Thank you to Robert A. Barnett, Food Editor, for his writing and editing of this book; and Holly Harper McPeak, Nutrition Program Coordinator, for her energy in supervising the recipe development and working with the chefs.

Thank you to Nutrition and Technical Services Division; Office of Analysis and Evaluation; Cooperative State Research, Education and Extension Service; Agricultural Marketing Service; the Department's Design Center, Printing Division and Office of Communications; FCS Public Information Office; and the Dietary Guidance Working Group for all their input and assistance. And to Linda Ebert, and Renee Prioleau of NTSD for reviewing the recipes and providing the nutrient analysis.

And this book would not have been possible without the clerical support of Gail Brown and Aggie Fitzgerald-Chab. Thank you to David Sutton and Julie Olson for the dynamic design of this book.

Thank you to the Culinary Institute of America for testing the recipes. Especially to Chef Ronald DeSantis, CMC, and his team of chefs, Martin Hopkins, Craig Edwards, Tonya Livingston, David Distenfeld, Joseph Krincek, Chris Boehme, Adam Bruce, Daniel Lestrid, and Thomas Giudice.

Many of the activities in this book come from the Scholastic Teacher Resource materials developed in cooperation with USDA's Team Nutrition.

A special thank you to the FCS Regional staff, State agencies, and the thousands of principals and school food service professionals across the country for teaming up to make school meals healthier, and to the families with children in the school meals programs for their efforts to eat more healthily at home.

Table of Contents

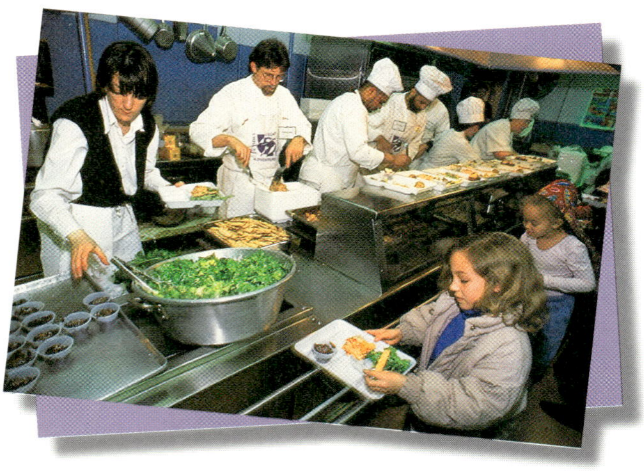

Introduction

About *Food, Family and Fun*

In communities across the country, families are taking steps to serve healthier meals at home. Now school meals will also be healthier and more appealing to your children. In fact, in June 1995 the Federal Government, recognizing its national health responsibility, made final a new policy ensuring that all school meals meet the *Dietary Guidelines for Americans*...that means school breakfasts and lunches will soon be lower in fat and sodium.

To help support the implementation of this new rule, the United States Department of Agriculture created Team Nutrition. Its mission is to improve the health and education of children. It does so by creating innovative public and private partnerships that promote food choices for a healthful diet through the media, schools, families, and the community.

Team Nutrition involves children and their families in nutrition education activities in the classroom, cafeteria, community, and at home. It also provides school food service staff with training, recipes, and resource materials to help them serve healthier meals.

Food, Family and Fun has been produced by Team Nutrition to help you provide healthful, affordable meals at home, and to answer your children's questions about food and health in fun and entertaining ways.

We asked parents just like you what they would look for in a book like this. They told us they wanted easy-to-use recipes that could provide families with nutrition information. They also wanted fun activities that could help them learn with their children about healthful eating.

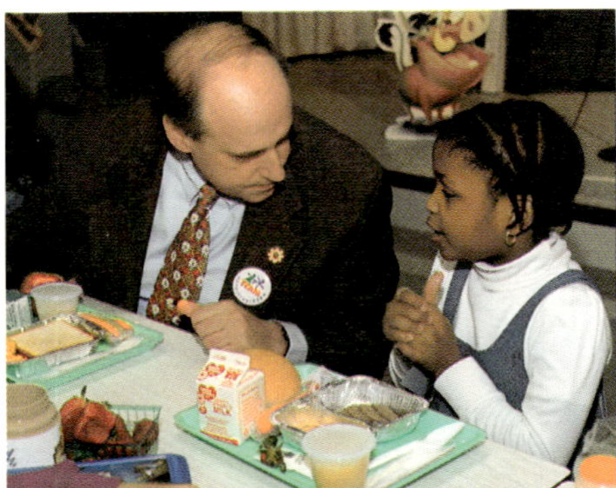

Secretary of Agriculture Dan Glickman says, "Nothing is more important than our children. And for 50 years, the National School Lunch Program has played a vitally important role in promoting their good health and education with nutritious meals at school. As the program gears up for the next 50 years, we're reaching out to families — the most important influence on children's diets — to ensure that better meals at school go hand-in-hand with healthy eating at home."

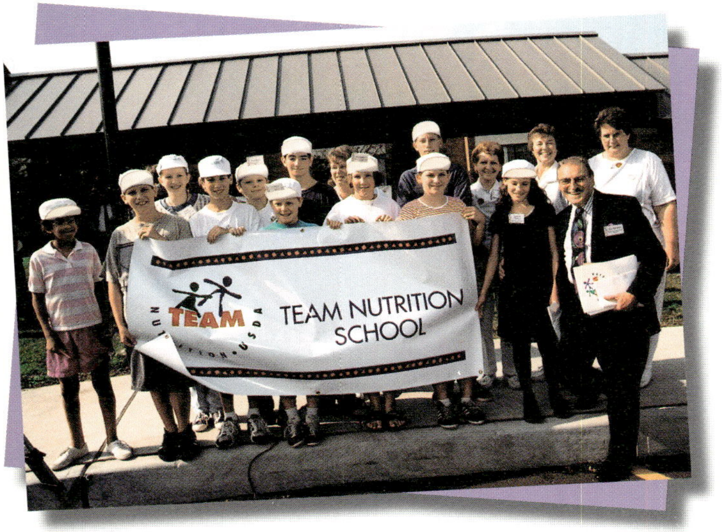

This book is also filled with recipes from some of the nation's top chefs who have volunteered their time to bring you seasonal and healthy ideas for making easy, affordable, and delicious dishes at home with your children's help. There are also learning activities you can do with your children both at home and at school and fun facts to read together. We've also included a comprehensive Resources section (*see pg 78*) to give you helpful information—from where to find farmers' markets in your area, to a listing of local cooperative extension specialists, to where to call or write for more nutrition information, and how to read a food label.

This year the USDA has provided new recipes to all schools in the National School Lunch Program. Some of those recipes are featured in this collection. Yes, you too can prepare some of the recipes your children will be served that are lower in fat and meet the U.S. Dietary Guidelines. Healthy eating does start at home.

We want Team Nutrition to help your entire family eat more healthfully.

What Parents Can Do

You are part of this historic change — the most important part. Good nutrition begins at home — and should continue at school. But it takes more than rules to make healthful school meals and to reach our goal of healthy children. To improve our children's school lunches, parents need to get involved in their schools.

That's why we created **Team Nutrition.** It is a network of public and private partnerships of parents, teachers, food service staff, health and education groups, and the food and agricultural community. These partnerships come together at the community level through the Team Nutrition Schools program.

Thousands and thousands of Team Nutrition Schools are leading the way in improving the school meals locally. At Team Nutrition Schools, a coalition of community volunteers is dedicated to making the school lunch program better, and to providing fun and entertaining nutrition education activities in the classroom and the cafeteria. Students in Team Nutrition Schools bring parent materials home, to link school learning with nutrition education activities that can be shared with the family.

How To Use This Book

To commemorate the 50th anniversary of the National School Lunch Program, this book contains 50 lower fat, low-cost recipes for families. And to reflect how what we eat changes with the seasons, it is divided into the 12 months of the year.

Each month contains 4 to 5 easy-to-use recipes. There are main dishes, side dishes, desserts, and snacks. In some cases, you can combine all the recipes together to make a meal. For other months, the recipes stand alone.

To help achieve balanced nutrition, taste, and economy, we have emphasized seasonal ingredients. For example, in the winter, winter squash is least expensive (and tastes best!) while tomatoes are cheaper and most delicious in the summer.

Some foods, such as citrus fruits (oranges, grapefruits), are least expensive in a particular season (winter), but available all year round. So while we emphasize them in the winter, we also use them throughout the year. Other foods, such as canned and frozen items, poultry, fish, lowfat beef and pork, beans, and dairy foods, are available all the time.

Finding Out About Foods Throughout the Seasons

In each season, we emphasize eight themes. Each theme provides nutrition activities for family learning and fun. Here are the themes:

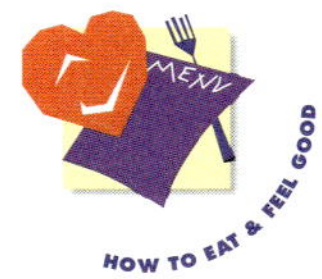

Nutrition, or *"How to Eat to Feel Good."* These are action items, and nutrition activities that relate to food and health.

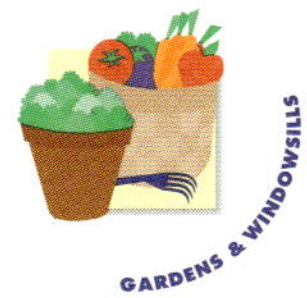

Agriculture, or *"Gardens and Windowsills."* We'll show you how to teach your children to grow foods on kitchen windowsills, or in the backyard — and how to get closer to affordable, seasonal foods that are grown in your community.

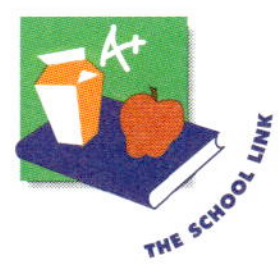

Education, or *"The School Link."* These are activities that relate to what your child may be learning in school as part of Team Nutrition activities.

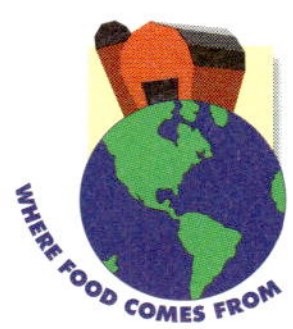

Food Facts, or *"Where Food Comes From."* Food is a perfect way to teach your children about history, geography, and agriculture.

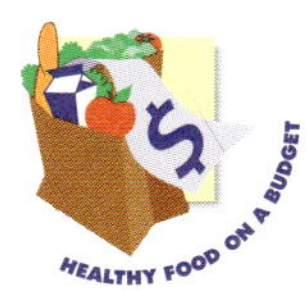

Practical Home Economics, or *"Healthy Food on a Budget."* These are suggestions to make shopping and cooking easier, to save money, and to plan. We'll share these.

Cooking Skill Education, or "***Children in the Kitchen***." Many children love to cook or prepare foods. One recipe each month is designed to involve children so they have fun making something good to eat.

Family Meals, or "***Families Eating Together***." Sharing meals is important. You know that it can be a special time for families to listen and learn from each other. These are some ideas about how to make family meals easier and more fun.

The recipe collection that follows also contains a sampling of **School Lunch Recipes** from USDA's New School Lunch and Breakfast Recipes, "A Tool Kit for Healthy School Meals."

Nutrition information is provided for each recipe. Optional ingredients are not included.

Food, Family and Fun — *Putting it into action*

__Team Nutrition__ is helping to ensure that your children are eating healthful meals at school and you are ensuring that your children are eating healthier meals at home. USDA recognizes the challenges that parents face in providing balanced meals for your family that taste good. We hope that this book, filled with seasonal recipes, community resources, and lots of family activities, will give you some tools to make it a little easier and more fun. As we commemorate the 50th anniversary of the National School Lunch Program together we leave you with one thought: Investing in your children's nutritional health today will make them your healthy adults tomorrow. Welcome to the team!!

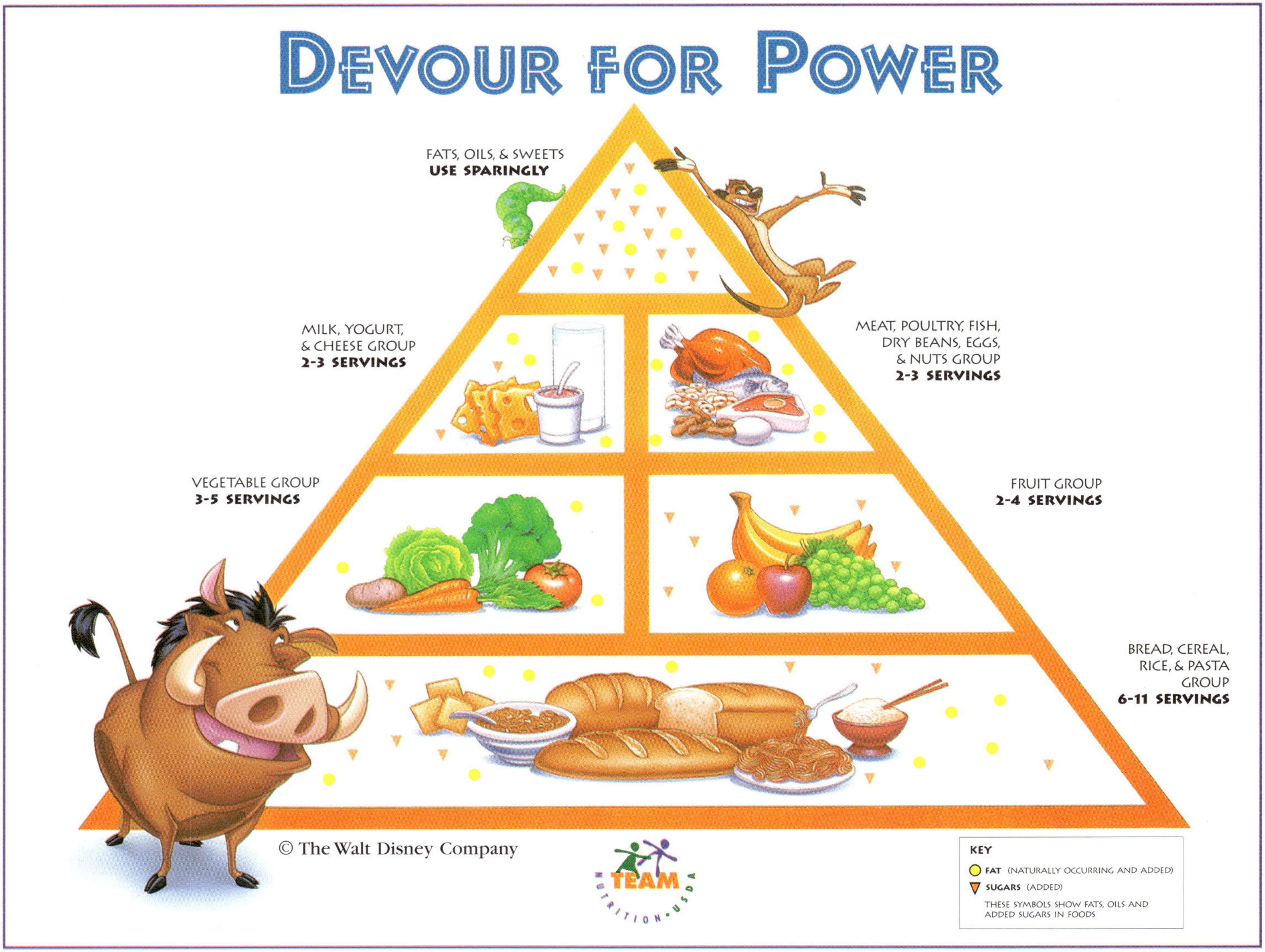

This graphic was developed as part of a cooperative relationship between the USDA's Team Nutrition and the Walt Disney Company.

What Is a Healthy Diet?

The following summarizes key concepts from the Dietary Guidelines for Americans, developed by the United States Departments of Agriculture and Health and Human Services, and contains the best, most up-to-date advice from nutrition scientists.

- ***Eat a variety of foods*** *to get the energy, protein, vitamins, minerals, and fiber you need for good health.*
- ***Balance the food you eat with physical activity; maintain or improve your weight*** *to reduce your chances of having high blood pressure, heart disease, a stroke, certain cancers, and the most common kind of diabetes.*
- ***Choose a diet with plenty of grain products, vegetables, and fruit*** *which are important sources of fiber, complex carbohydrates, and other food components that can help reduce your risk of some chronic diseases.*
- ***Choose a diet low in fat, saturated fat, and cholesterol*** *to reduce your risk of heart disease and certain cancers, and to help you maintain a healthy weight. Because fat contains more than twice the calories of an equal amount of carbohydrates or protein, a diet low in fat can help maintain healthy weight.*
- ***Choose a diet moderate in sugars*** *A diet with lots of sugars often has foods with too many calories and too few nutrients and can contribute to tooth decay and overweight.*
- ***Choose a diet moderate in salt and sodium*** *which may help reduce the risk of high blood pressure.*
- ***If you drink alcoholic beverages, do so in moderation*** *because alcoholic beverages supply calories but little or no nutrients and in excess are harmful. Children and adolescents should not drink at all.*

Unfortunately, most children do not consume a diet that meets the Dietary Guidelines outlined above. Less than one in five children eat the recommended numbers of servings of fruit and vegetables daily. Team Nutrition needs you to join in and help kids make food choices for a healthy diet.

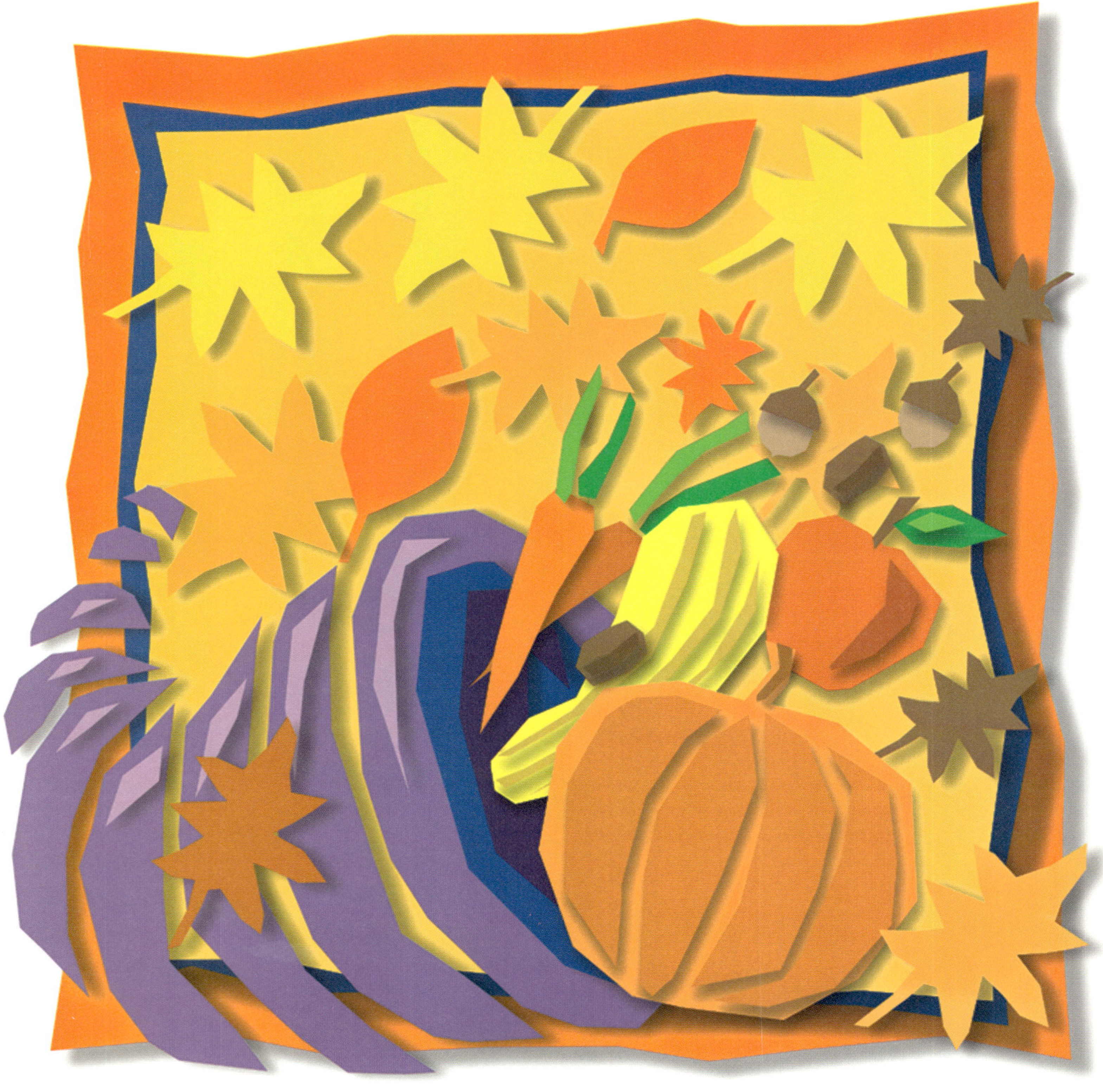

Autumn

Autumn, or fall, is the season of harvest. Across the country, farmers are bringing in their crops. So are gardeners. In many parts of the country, fall blankets the countryside foliage with brilliant reds, oranges and yellows.

In supermarkets and the farmers' markets, the best of the season's bounty is on display. In September, summer fruits and vegetables, including tomatoes, summer squash, and peppers are still available. By October, the month that ends with Halloween, pumpkins and winter squash, such as acorn and Hubbard, begin to appear. They are inexpensive and very nutritious. Crisp fall apples come into season; potatoes and sweet potatoes arrive. By November, we celebrate our national

Autumn Chef Teams Included:

Michael Romano, Tom Colicchio, Alan Harding, Alan Tardi, Nora Pouillon, Carole Wagner, Randall Warder, Cass Peterson, Stacey FitzSimmons, and Jeffrey Tomchek.

bounty with Thanksgiving, when we eat harvest foods and turkey, join together, and give thanks for the season's gifts to the kitchen.

In Season:

Vegetables:
Brussels sprouts, cabbage, cucumbers, eggplant, lima beans, onions, okra, peppers, potatoes, sweet corn, sweet potatoes, summer, squash, tomatoes, winter squash.

Fruits:
Apples, avocado, cantaloupe, dates, figs, grapes, honeydew melons, lemons, peaches, pears, plums, prunes, Valencia oranges.

Also,
Tree nuts such as almonds and walnuts; many fish and shellfish (including oysters), all meats, poultry, and dairy products.

September is also the beginning of a new school year in most areas. This year school children will be enjoying new, more healthful, tastier school meals. They will be learning about how food is produced, how it affects their bodies, and how to make better food choices to stay healthy.

The recipes that appear on the following pages take full advantage of the foods that are at their peak in the fall. You'll find every food group in the Food Guide Pyramid (pg 79) represented here: Bread, Cereal, Rice and Pasta; Fruits; Vegetables; Milk, Yogurt and Cheese; and Meat, Poultry, Fish, Dry Beans, Eggs and Nuts. In September, we take advantage of still-available tomatoes and summer squash in a casserole (pg 16), dip fresh string beans in a yogurt dip (pg 17), and invite our children to help us "skewer" fresh fruit kabobs in chocolate sauce (pg 18). In October, we pair pork chops with apples (pg 19), and make a meal out of a potato (pg 20). And in November, we bake beans in the New England style (pg 24).

Have a fun Fall!

Baked Lemon Chicken

30 minutes Serves: 5

Your children will like this! The lemon slices on these chicken pieces look like circus wheels. Ask your child to help you top the chicken with the lemon slices before it goes into the oven.

- **1** 3½ pound chicken, skinned, cut into 10 pieces
- **¼** tsp salt
- **¼** tsp pepper
- **1½** thinly sliced garlic cloves (or 1 tsp. garlic powder)
- **4** fresh thyme sprigs (or 1 tsp dried thyme)
- **3** cups thinly-sliced onions
- **1½** cups chicken stock or water
- **¼** cup lemon juice
- **1** lemon, sliced into 10 slices, seeds removed

1. **Combine** salt, pepper, garlic, and thyme.
2. **Lay** chicken pieces into a 11″ x 13″ baking pan. **Sprinkle** seasonings over chicken.
3. **Combine** onions, stock, and lemon juice in a sauce pan. **Heat** to a boil.
4. **Pour** hot lemon mixture around chicken. **Top** each chicken piece with a lemon slice.
5. **Bake** for 30 minutes at 400°F. until golden brown and juices are clear colored.

Nutrients per serving
2 pieces

Calories	253	Saturated Fat	2.4 g	Iron	2.1 mg
Protein	34 g	Cholesterol	101 mg	Calcium	53 mg
Carbohydrate	10 g	Vitamin A	20 RE	Sodium	219 mg
Total Fat	8.7 g	Vitamin C	27 mg	Dietary Fiber	2 g

HOW TO EAT TO FEEL GOOD

Are you eating 3-5 vegetables a day? If you aren't, a few small changes can improve your diet. The Food Guide Pyramid can help you choose a more healthful diet for your family. Having a vegetable juice or adding a vegetable for a snack each day can make a big difference in your diet.

Tomato, Squash and Onion Casserole

25–30 minutes Serves: 8

In September, tomatoes and yellow squash are in season. That means they are the most affordable and the most delicious. This dish is good served hot.

- **1** Tbsp olive oil
- **2** tsp minced garlic
- **3** small onions, sliced
- **1** tsp salt
- **½** tsp freshly-ground pepper
- **1** Tbsp each fresh thyme, oregano and basil (or 1 tsp each, dried)
- **1** medium zucchini, washed, cut into thin slices (about ½ pound)
- **1** medium yellow squash, washed, cut into thin slices (about ½ pound)
- **6** fresh plum tomatoes, cut into medium slices

Preheat oven to 400° F.

1. **Saute** onions and garlic in 1 Tbsp oil over medium heat, until onions are tender and browned. **Place** in oven-proof dish and **season** with half the salt, pepper and herbs.
2. **Arrange** zucchini on top of onions, then place a layer of yellow squash next with a layer of tomatoes. **Sprinkle** with rest of herbs, salt, and pepper.
3. **Bake**, covered, for 25-30 minutes.

Nutrients per serving
1 cup

Calories	56	Saturated Fat	.3 g	Iron	1.1 mg
Protein	2 g	Cholesterol	0 mg	Calcium	31 mg
Carbohydrate	9 g	Vitamin A	80 RE	Sodium	301 mg
Total Fat	2.2 g	Vitamin C	25 mg	Dietary Fiber	3 g

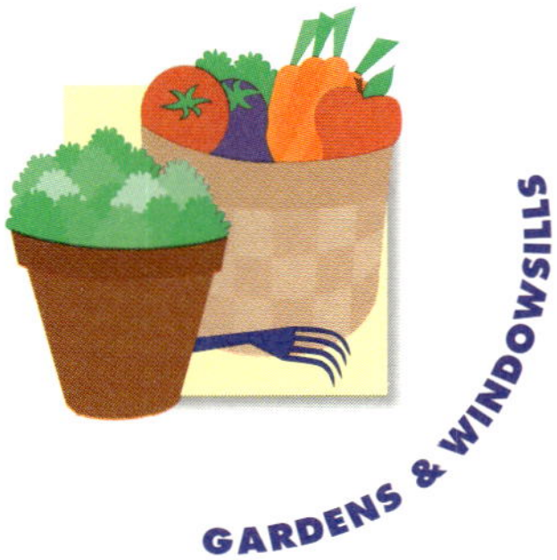

Fall is a great time of year to take a trip to a farm stand, local farmers' market or farm. Try new varieties of squash or pumpkins. Go apple picking at a farm or choose your apples at a market and try different types.

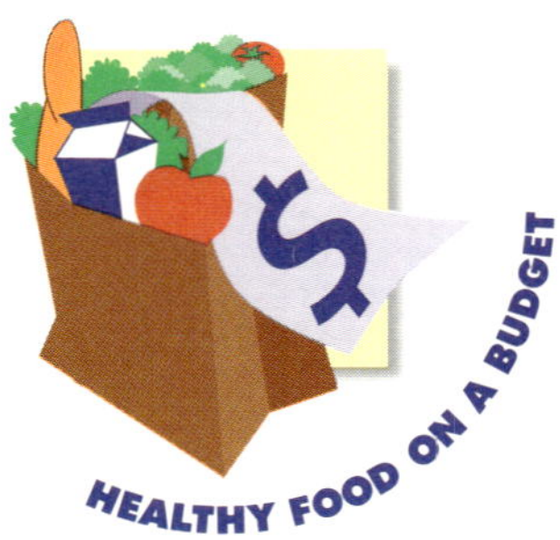

If you go to a farmers' market this month, the early bird gets the freshest food. But if you go late in the day, in the late afternoon, you may get some real bargains. The farmers would rather sell their fruits and vegetables than have to truck them back home.

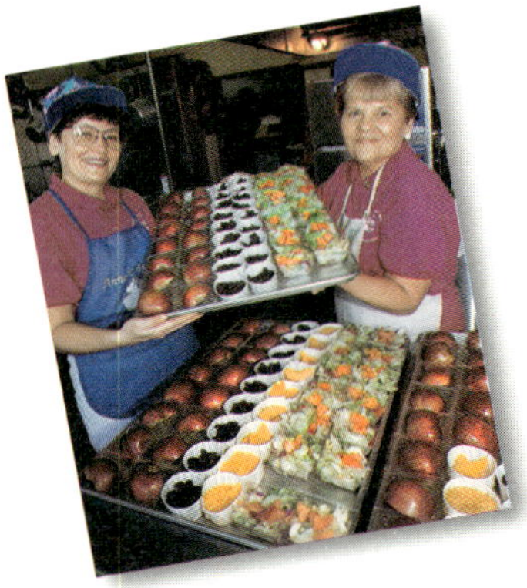

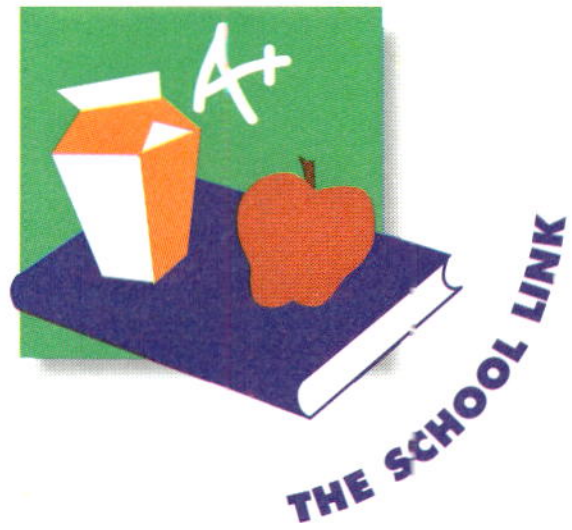

Is a tomato a fru t or a vegetable? The surprising answer: tomatoes are fruits that are usually called vegetables. Most fruits have seeds. Fruits are usually eaten raw, while many vegetables are cooked. Here's a game: Ask your child to name as many vegetables as possible in three minutes. Count how many different vegetables were served this week at school.

Yogurt-Mustard Dip

10 minutes Serves: 8

Here's an easy snack with fresh vegetables and nonfat yogurt.

- **1** Tbsp chopped onion
- **2** Tbsp chopped sweet pickle (or relish)
- **2** Tbsp chopped fresh parsley (or fresh dill), use half as much for dried
- **1** Tbsp prepared mustard
- **½** tsp paprika (optional—if you like a pink color)
- **1** cup nonfat plain yogurt
- **1** lb vegetables, raw or lightly steamed, any combination: green beans, cauliflower or broccoli florets (cut into small pieces), carrots (peeled and cut into sticks)

1. **Combine** together onion, pickle, parsley, mustard, and paprika (optional).
2. **Mix** into yogurt.
3. **Put** dip in a small bowl in the middle of a large plate. **Surround** it with vegetables for dipping. **Serve.**

For a taste variation, try Curry Dip: Substitute 2 tsp of curry powder for the mustard, add 1 Tbsp milk, and ⅛ tsp of sugar. Add 1 to 2 Tbsp raisins (optional).

Nutrients per serving (Dip only)
2 Tbsp

Calories	22	Saturated Fat	.0 g	Iron	.1 mg
Protein	2 g	Cholesterol	0 mg	Calcium	64 mg
Carbohydrate	3 g	Vitamin A	5 RE	Sodium	70 mg
Total Fat	.2 g	Vitamin C	2 mg	Dietary Fiber	0 g

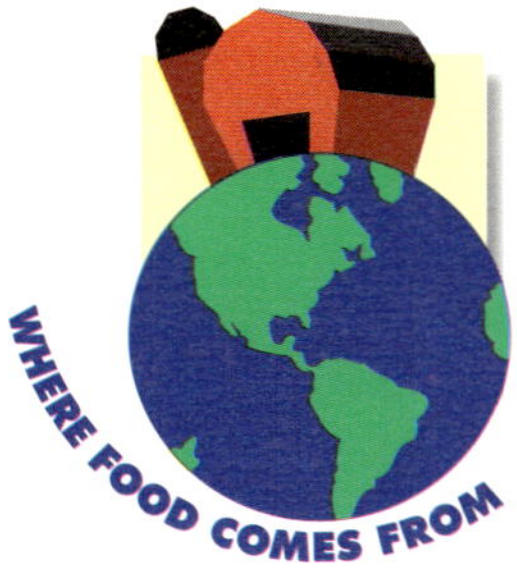

Where do vegetables come from? Some grow on bushes, while many vegetables grow on vines or, sometimes, underground, like carrots and potatoes. But all vegetables come from seeds. Inside are the seeds that could grow new plants. Some are easy to find, such as squash, beans, and eggplant.

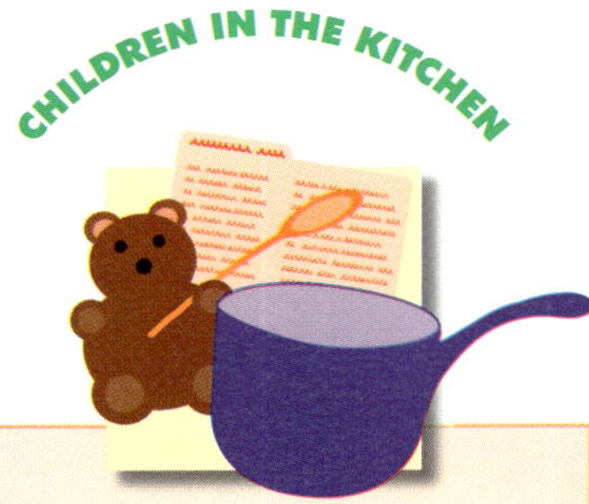

Fresh Fruit Kabobs with Chocolate Sauce

5 minutes Serves: 6

This is fun party food, or dessert after dinner. You can serve it soon after making it, or make it, then refrigerate.

- **12** strawberries
- **24** melon balls (honeydew, cantaloupe)
- **6** ounces angel food cake, cut into 1-inch cubes
- **6** marshmallows
- **1⅓** cups semi-sweet chocolate chips
- **1** Tbsp lowfat buttermilk (or lowfat milk)
- **6** wooden skewers

1. Have kids **wash** strawberries, **picking** off stems. With a melon baller or a small spoon, have them **make** melon balls. Carefully! If kids can handle a knife, have them **cut** cake into squares.
2. Have kids **arrange** fruit and cake on wooden skewers. The pattern is up to them! **Place** skewered fruit sticks on a serving plate.
3. The adult **melts** chocolate chips and milk together over low heat.
4. Together **pour** sauce over fruit sticks, turning over to cover. Let cool a moment. Serve to hungry kids!

Nutrients per serving
1 kabob

Calories	354	Saturated Fat	7 g	Iron	2.1 mg
Protein	5 g	Cholesterol	0 mg	Calcium	96 mg
Carbohydrate	63 g	Vitamin A	98 RE	Sodium	251 mg
Total Fat	12.6 g	Vitamin C	99 mg	Dietary Fiber	7 g

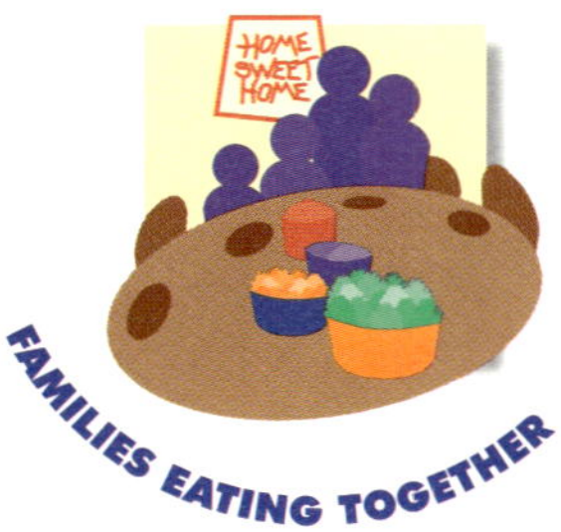

Throw a Sense-sational Tasting Party. As a family, work together to plan tasting events. Choose different vegetables that can be eaten raw, such as carrots, broccoli, celery, cauliflower, and zucchini sticks. Have children describe each food, using words to describe its taste, how it feels in their mouth, and how it sounds when they chew!

Pork Chops with Apples

10 minutes Serves: 4

If you like a sweeter apple, use a Macintosh. If you like a tart taste, use Granny Smith. Apples are good sources of fiber. Serve with rice, and a steamed green vegetable or a crunchy green salad — or both!

If you would prefer, bake pork chops in a 350°F oven for 25 minutes instead of cooking on top of range. Using a skillet is faster, but use vegetable oil!

- **4** small apples
- **4** pork chops, ½ -inch thick, trimmed of all fat
- vegetable oil spray
- **¼** tsp salt and ⅛ tsp pepper (optional)
- **1** Tbsp vegetable oil

1. **Core** apples and **cut** into quarters. Then **cut** each quarter into 3–4 slices.
2. **Heat** a non-stick skillet over medium heat. If non-stick skillet is not available, **spray** with vegetable spray. **Place** chops in the pan and **brown** on both sides for 3-5 minutes. **Salt and pepper** the pork chops (optional).
3. **Push** pork chops to the center of the skillet. **Place** apples around chops. **Drizzle** oil over the top of apples. **Cook** for 5 minutes, **shaking** the pan from time to time and **turning** the apple slices over to **brown** both sides.
4. **Remove** chops from pan to a serving plate; **surround** with the apples.

Nutrients per serving
1 chop, ½ cup apples

Calories	250	Saturated Fat	3.0 g	Iron	.9 mg
Protein	19 g	Cholesterol	52 mg	Calcium	20 mg
Carbohydrate	21 g	Vitamin A	8 RE	Sodium	42 mg
Total Fat	10.4 g	Vitamin C	8 mg	Dietary Fiber	4 g

HOW TO EAT TO FEEL GOOD

Achieve the goal of "eating a variety of food" by eating the number of recommended servings in the Food Pyramid. How? Have each family member keep a list of foods eaten for 2 days. Everyone writes down each food, and the amount eaten throughout the day. Then, count up how many different foods from each food group were eaten each day. Compare to the Food Guide Pyramid.

THE SCHOOL LINK

This month includes United Nations Day (October 24). Why not create an "Adventures in Eating" bulletin board at home? Put a map of the world on it. Get colored pins. Each time a child tries foods from each Pyramid Food Group they make a colorful cutout of the food, and attach it to the map with a pin, in the area of the world where that food is commonly eaten. Remember to celebrate "National School Lunch Week."

Meal in a Potato

45 minutes - 1 hour Serves 4

This makes a fun side dish or hearty snack. To make it into a true meal, add leftover meat, poultry, fish, or mashed beans, and vegetables like chopped spinach or broccoli to the potato.

If you have a child who is older and helps to get dinner started, this is a nice recipe to suggest. (To save on time: "bake" the potatoes in a microwave.)

4 large potatoes
1 Tbsp oil
4 Tbsp grated lowfat cheese (mozzarella or cheddar)
¼ tsp salt
⅛ tsp pepper
⅛ tsp of nutmeg

1. **Preheat** oven to 425° F. **Scrub** potatoes well. **Dry** with a towel. **Rub** the outside with oil. **Bake** about 45 minutes - 1 hour until potato is soft.
2. **Cut** off a cap lengthwise. **Scoop** out some of the pulp and mix with the cheese, salt, pepper, and nutmeg. **Spoon** back into potato. **Replace** cap. **Serve**.

Nutrients per serving
1 potato

Calories	262	Saturated Fat	.9 g	Iron	2.8 mg
Protein	6 g	Cholesterol	1 mg	Calcium	50 mg
Carbohydrate	51 g	Vitamin A	4 RE	Sodium	204 mg
Total Fat	4.1 g	Vitamin C	26 mg	Dietary Fiber	5 g

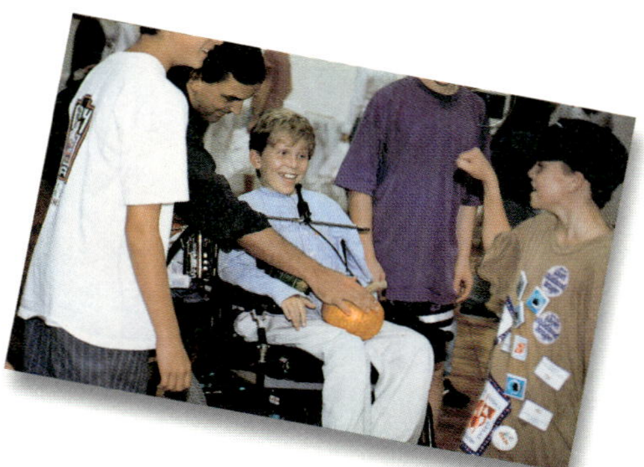

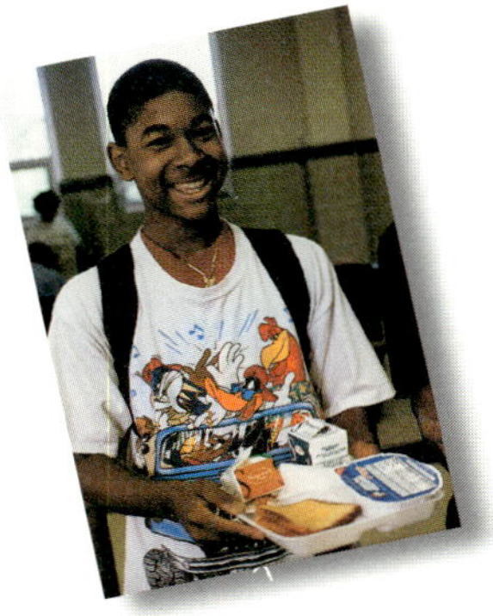

Fruit Cole Slaw

15 minutes Serves: 6

This makes a nice side dish for lunch or snack, and it's fabulous at picnics and barbecues.

- ½ head of cabbage shredded (approximately 2 quarts)
- **1** 16 oz can fruit cocktail, juice-packed, drained
- **1** cup nonfat plain yogurt
- Juice of **1** lemon (or 2 limes)
- ½ cup honey
- ¼ cup vinegar
- **1** banana, sliced
- ½ tsp salt
- ⅛ tsp pepper
- **3** Tbsp sliced and toasted almonds (optional)

1. **Shred** cabbage.
2. **Combine** all ingredients in a large bowl.
3. **Top** with almonds (optional) and **enjoy!**

Nutrients per serving
½ cup

Calories	185	Saturated Fat	.1 g	Iron	.9 mg
Protein	4 g	Cholesterol	0 mg	Calcium	125 mg
Carbohydrate	46 g	Vitamin A	33 RE	Sodium	244 mg
Total Fat	.4 g	Vitamin C	31 mg	Dietary Fiber	3 g

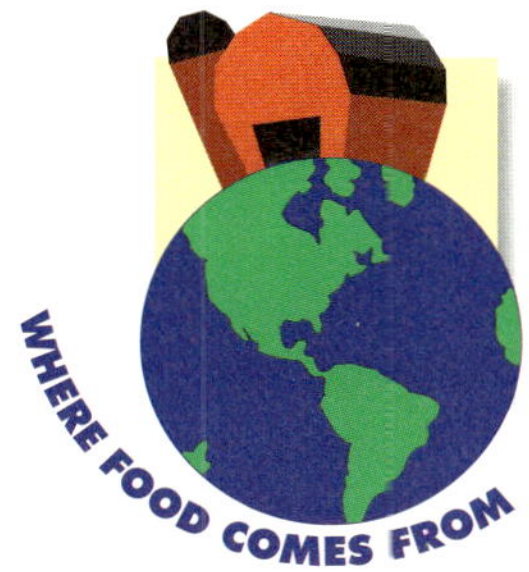

The official date of Columbus Day is on October 12th. When Christopher Columbus first came to the Americas, Native Americans were eating foods no others had ever seen: pumpkins, squash, corn, tomatoes, potatoes. Imagine that — Italy without tomatoes or the Irish without potatoes. Thai food without hot chile peppers! But it was true. Native American foods soon traveled around the world, and became popular. Your children can look up Columbus in the library, and write down all the foods that were native to America, but soon traveled all around the world.

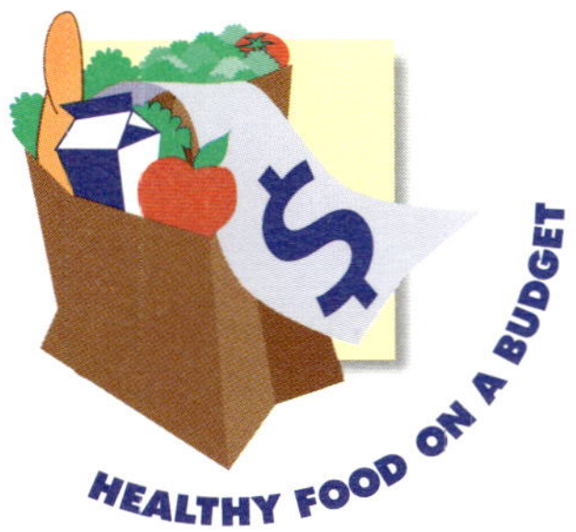

Spruce up old favorites by adding new ingredients. Include fruits, vegetables or extra grains in recipes that may not call for them. Add diced carrots to rice. Add fruit to meat dishes, like sliced apples to pork dishes. Sliced bananas and shredded carrots on sandwiches make a tasty difference. Try a meatless dinner once or twice a week. Beans, dry or canned, provide plenty of protein for a family, as well as vitamins and minerals.

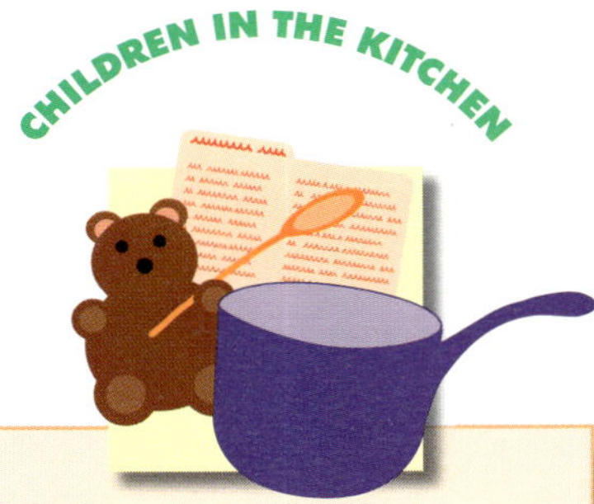

Crunchy Pumpkin Seeds

About 20 minutes
Serves: Depends on how big a pumpkin you have!

It's fun to make a scary Halloween pumpkin, and it's fun to toast the seeds and eat them. Seeds contain everything needed to grow a new pumpkin, and are a tasty snack, too!

Seeds from 1 Halloween Pumpkin
1 tsp salt per 1 cup of seeds

Preheat oven to 350°F.

1. Have the kids help **carve** the Halloween pumpkin. When they scoop out the inside pulp that contains the seeds, **reserve**.
2. Have kids stand at the sink (use a stool if they are too low). **Put** pulp in a colander. Have kids **wash** pulp and stringy matter off seeds under cold running water. **Blot** seeds dry with a clean cloth or paper towel.
3. Have kids **spread** seeds out on a cookie sheet. The seeds should be in a single layer, and they shouldn't touch each other!
4. **Sprinkle** the seeds with just a little salt. An adult **puts** the tray in the oven.
5. **Check** the seeds after 12 minutes. They are done when they are dry and light brown. How long this will take depends on how many there are, and how dry they are when they go in the oven.
6. Let **cool** before eating!

Nutrients per serving
2 Tbsp

Calories	148	Saturated Fat	2.3 g	Iron	4.2 mg
Protein	9 g	Cholesterol	0 mg	Calcium	12 mg
Carbohydrate	4 g	Vitamin A	10 RE	Sodium	295 mg
Total Fat	12.0 g	Vitamin C	1 mg	Dietary Fiber	1 g

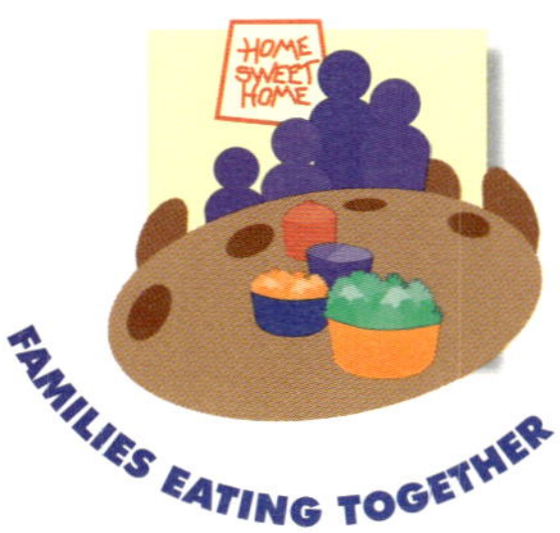

Create a meal based on the ethnic heritage of grandparents; ask for recipes. Shop with an older family member or neighbor to buy the ingredients; prepare the foods your grandparent fixed for your parents. Make a cookbook of family recipes.

Turkey-Topped Pizza

10 minutes   Serves: 8

You can add any of these to the top of your pizza: thin slices of green pepper, yellow pepper, or red pepper; fresh basil leaves or oregano; thin slices of red onion, yellow onion, or Spanish onion; grilled eggplant, zucchini, broccoli florets; mushroom slices; and any kind of olives.

- **9** oz ground turkey
- **½** tsp olive oil
- **1** Tbsp garlic powder (or 1-2 fresh garlic cloves, minced)
- **1** Tbsp onion powder
- **1** tsp fennel seed
- **¼** tsp dried oregano leaves
- **¼** tsp Italian seasoning (optional)
- **2** whole wheat English muffins, split
- **4** pita bread
- **2** cups Garden Fresh Tomato Sauce (*see pg 86*)
- **9** oz lowfat mozzarella cheese, shredded

1. In a hot skillet, **add** oil, ground turkey and all other seasonings.
2. **Cook** until turkey resembles a finely ground mixture and temperature is 165°F and juices are clear-colored.
3. **Place** muffin halves and pitas on sheet pan. **Divide** and **spread** turkey topping evenly over tops of muffin halves and pitas. **Top** with sauce, and sprinkle on mozzarella.
4. **Bake** in oven at 375°F until cheeses melt, about 5-10 minutes.

Variation: You can also use the turkey topping for other meals. Mix some into tomato sauce. Add ½ tsp of chili powder to season. Put in a taco shell— or hot dog bun — with shredded romaine lettuce.

Nutrients per serving
1 piece

Calories	218	Saturated Fat	3.1 g	Iron	1.7 mg
Protein	18 g	Cholesterol	34 mg	Calcium	298 mg
Carbohydrate	20 g	Vitamin A	60 RE	Sodium	377 mg
Total Fat	7.7 g	Vitamin C	7 mg	Dietary Fiber	3 g

Try more healthful ways of preparing meats, poultry and fish. Bake or broil rather than fry. Remove the skin from the poultry. Drain the fat. When using beef try leaner grades, such as USDA "Select."

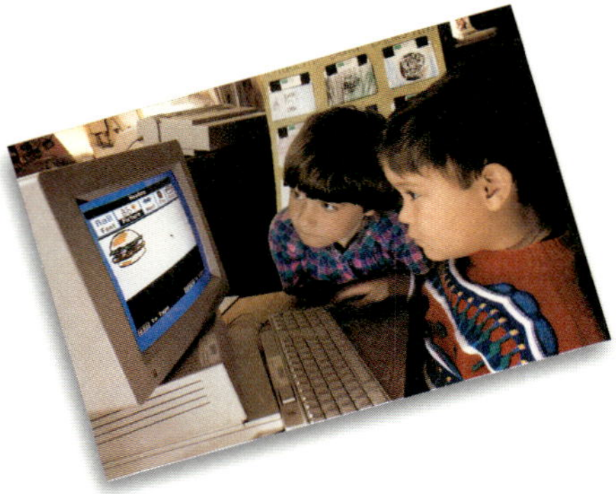

THE SCHOOL LINK

Have your children count how many servings from the meat group they had at school lunch this week. Remember, beans, eggs, nuts and peanut butter count in this group.

New England "Maple Baked Beans"

30 minutes or longer Serves: 6

2 12 oz cans vegetarian baked beans
½ cup maple-flavored syrup
⅓ cup onion, chopped
¼ cup catsup
1 Tbsp prepared mustard
¼ cup lowfat white cheddar cheese, shredded (optional)

Preheat oven to 350°F.

1. **Mix** all ingredients together. **Pour** into a greased casserole and **bake**, uncovered, for 30 minutes or longer.
2. **Sprinkle** cheddar (optional) on top for the last ten minutes of baking. **Serve** warm.

Nutrients per serving
½ cup

Calories	198	Saturated Fat	0.2 g	Iron	1.8 mg
Protein	6 g	Cholesterol	0 mg	Calcium	55 mg
Carbohydrate	46 g	Vitamin A	24 RE	Sodium	581 mg
Total Fat	0.8 g	Vitamin C	5 mg	Dietary Fiber	6 g

Three-Grain Pilaf

45 minutes Serves: 6

Orzo is pasta that looks like rice. Barley adds a nutty flavor. Together, with the rice, the three make an exciting grain dish.

1 medium onion, minced
½ cup peppers, green or red or both
1 oz vegetable oil (or butter)
½ cup golden raisins
¼ cup chopped fresh parsley
½ cup pearled barley
5 cups chicken broth (or water with one bouillon cube)
1 cup converted rice
½ cup dry orzo pasta
3 bay leaves
½ cup chopped nuts such as pine, almonds or walnuts (optional)
seasonings to taste

1. **Saute** onion and peppers in oil or butter for 5 minutes. **Remove** from heat. **Add** raisins and parsley; **set aside.**
2. **Cook** barley in 5 cups of stock or water for 20 minutes, covered, then **add** rice and and **cook** for 15 more minutes. **Add** orzo and bay leaves. **Cook** covered for another 5 minutes.
3. **Remove** bay leaves. **Fold in** sauteed vegetables and nuts (optional). **Add** seasonings (not too much salt!) **Serve.**

Nutrients per serving
1 cup

Calories	251	Saturated Fat	0.8 g	Iron	2.2 mg
Protein	8 g	Cholesterol	4 mg	Calcium	28 mg
Carbohydrate	46 g	Vitamin A	41 RE	Sodium	224 mg
Total Fat	4.0 g	Vitamin C	17 mg	Dietary Fiber	3 g

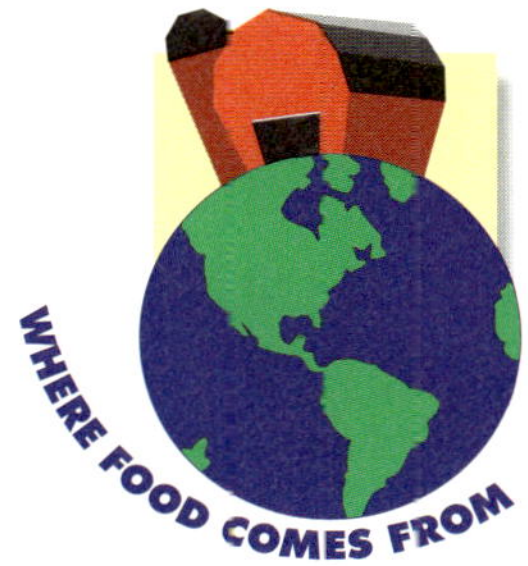

Visit a meat market, a fish market or a farm. Do you like to fish? Take your child.

HEALTHY FOOD ON A BUDGET

"Zip the Fat Off a Chicken". Before cooking, wash a whole (broiler) chicken. Put your hand between the skin and breast to loosen the skin. Do the same for the back and top of the drumsticks. Grab the loosened skin and pull off to "zip the skin" off the chicken. Use a knife to trim off any skin from the legs that did not pull off. Wash hands *after* handling the chicken and *before* handling any other foods.

Harvest Pumpkin Bread

1 hour Serves: 12

- **1** cup sugar
- ¼ cup margarine
- ¼ cup applesauce
- **2** eggs
- **1** cup (8 oz) solid pack pumpkin
- **2** cups all purpose flour
- ½ tsp salt
- **2** tsp baking powder
- ¼ tsp baking soda
- 1 tsp ground cinnamon
- ½ cup raisins
- 1 tsp grated orange rind
- ¼ cup orange juice
- ½ cup walnuts, chopped (optional)

Preheat oven to 350°F.

1. Lightly grease a 9″ x 5″ x 3″ loaf pan or coat with vegetable spray.
2. **Beat** sugar, margarine, and applesauce until creamy and light (about 5 minutes). **Add** eggs one at a time and continue to beat. **Add** pumpkin and mix until smooth.
3. **Combine** flour, salt, baking powder, baking soda, and cinnamon. **Stir** into pumpkin mixture and **mix** until smooth.
4. **Add** raisins, orange rind, orange juice and nuts (optional). **Stir** well and **pour** into loaf pan.
5. **Bake** at 350°F for 60-65 minutes. You can **test** doneness by sticking a wooden pick into loaf. If it **comes out** clean, loaf is done. Cut into 12 slices

Nutrients per serving
1 slice

Calories	220	Saturated Fat	0.9 g	Iron	1.7 mg
Protein	3.7 g	Cholesterol	35 mg	Calcium	65 mg
Carbohydrate	42 g	Vitamin A	513 RE	Sodium	261 mg
Total Fat	4.9 g	Vitamin C	3 mg	Dietary Fiber	2 g

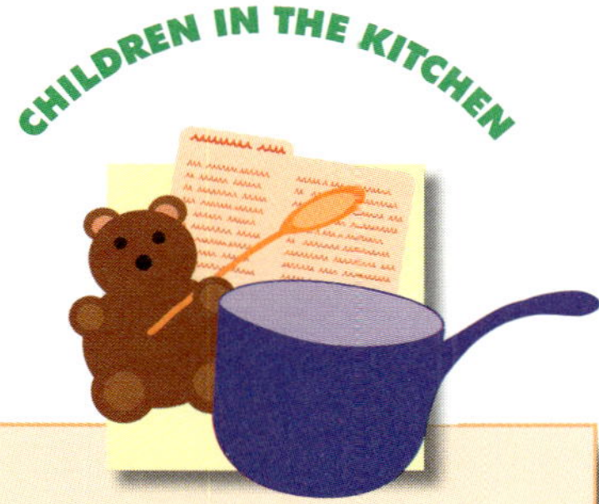

Baked Bananas

20 minutes Serves: 4

Here's a quiz for kids: How many bananas do eight halves make?

¼ cup brown sugar
¼ cup honey
2 Tbsp water
4 bananas

Preheat oven to 375°F.

1. In a pot, the adult **heats** brown sugar, honey and water over low heat for 5 minutes, until sugar dissolves.
2. Kids **peel** each banana, and **cut** each one in half, cross-wise. (That's *not* the long way, but right across the middle.) Kids **place** all 8 halves in a 9" x 12" baking pan. Kids carefully **pour** syrup over bananas.
3. Adult **puts** pan in oven. Bake for 5–10 minutes. Remove from oven, and turn bananas over. Bake 5–10 more minutes until slightly browned. **Remove** from oven.
4. To **serve,** kids carefully **take** each banana half out of pan, and **put** two halves onto each plate. Be very, very careful not to burn yourself! Adult **pours** syrup from baking pan into little pitcher. Kids **pour** syrup over each banana half. Everybody gets to **enjoy** dessert.

Nutrients per serving
2 halves

Calories	202	Saturated Fat	.2 g	Iron	.6 mg
Protein	1 g	Cholesterol	0 mg	Calcium	15 mg
Carbohydrate	53 g	Vitamin A	9 RE	Sodium	5 mg
Total Fat	.6 g	Vitamin C	10 mg	Dietary Fiber	3 g

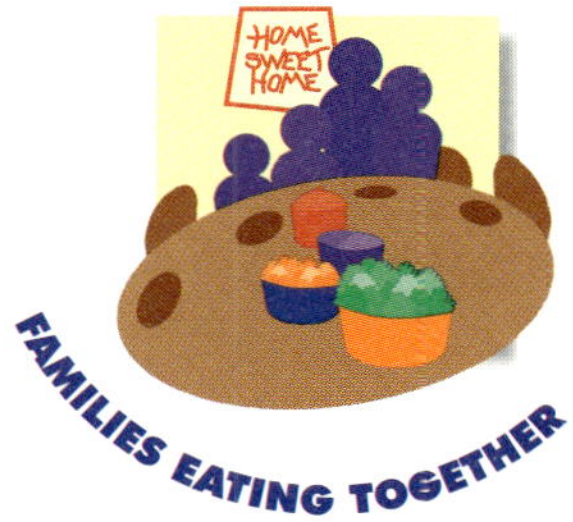

Thanksgiving is a unique American national holiday. It's an opportunity for families, including many generations, to sit down and celebrate together. Turkey is the favorite meat at this meal. Try using turkey leftovers in lowfat ways.

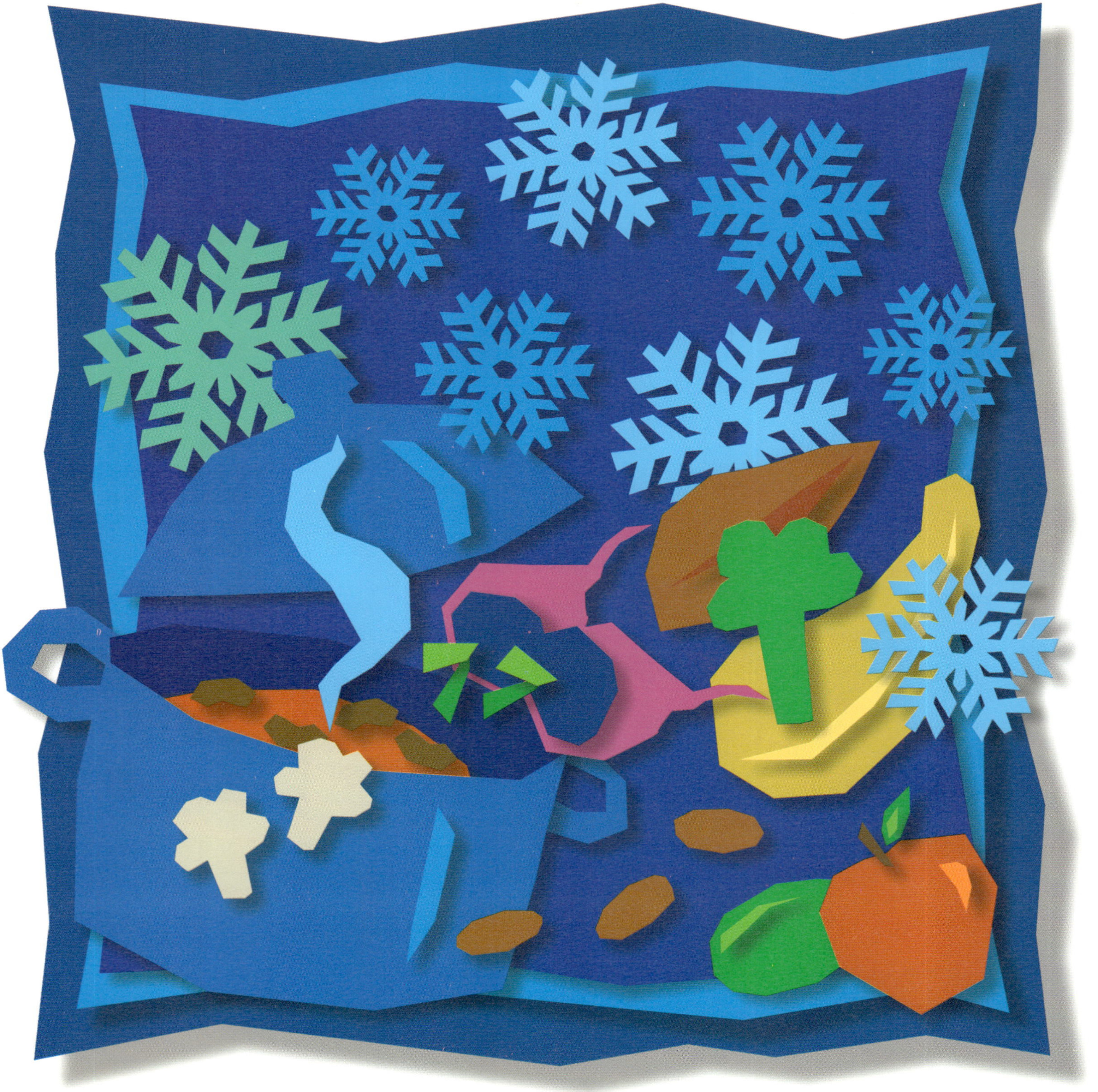

Winter

Winter is the coldest season of the year. In many parts of the country, snow blankets the ground and very little grows. It is not as easy to purchase seasonal vegetables and fruits as it is in the summer and fall, when gardens blossom. But there are still many seasonal foods that are inexpensive and nutritious. And, of course, frozen and canned fruits and vegetables, meats, fish and poultry products give ready access to many seasonal foods year round.

Some foods aren't affected by the seasons. The foundation of the Food Guide Pyramid — the Bread, Cereal, Rice, and Pasta Group — is available year round. So are the Milk, Yogurt, and Cheese Group and the Meat, Poultry, Fish, Dry Beans, Eggs, and Nuts Group.

Even in fruits, and in vegetables, there are many seasonal bargains. Citrus fruits, grown

Winter Chef Teams Included:

Robert Del Grande, Susan Spicer, Alice Waters, Alan Tangren, Marion Cunningham, Niloufer Ishaporia, Catherine Brandel, Rick Bayless and Deanne Bayless.

in southern parts of the country, are in peak season in the winter. These include grapefruit, navel oranges, and lemons. They are very good sources of Vitamin C. For an unusual taste treat, try our Oranges in Tangerine Juice (pg 33). Apples harvested in the autumn, are still available at a good price, as are winter pears.

Winter vegetables are as hardy as the season. Nutritious potatoes are firm and well-priced. So are sweet potatoes (see Sweet Potatoes with Lime, pg 39) and carrots. Cabbage-family vegetables, which include all kinds of cabbage, broccoli, brussels sprouts and cauliflower, are in peak season. These are also very nutritious. So are winter squash - that orange or red color is the color of beta-carotene, which the body converts to Vitamin A.

When we take advantage of the fruits and vegetables that are in peak season in the winter, we can eat according to the Food Guide Pyramid, with delicious foods that are within our budget.

In Season:

Vegetables: Beets, broccoli, brussels sprouts, cabbage, carrots, cauliflower, celery, potatoes, spinach, sweet potatoes, winter squash.

Fruits: Apples, avocado, dates, grapefruit, lemons, navel oranges, winter pears.

Also, Walnuts, all dairy, meat and poultry products, most fish and shellfish.

School Lunch Recipe

Baked Cajun Fish

25 minutes Serves: 6

- **6** white fish portions, 3-oz each (if frozen, thaw first in refrigerator)
- **1** Tbsp lemon juice
- **1½** Tbsp margarine or butter, melted

Seasonings:

- ¼ tsp paprika
- ½ tsp granulated garlic
- ¼ tsp onion powder
- ⅛ tsp white pepper
- ⅛ tsp ground oregano
- ⅛ tsp ground thyme

Preheat oven to 350°F.

1. In a small bowl, **combine** paprika, garlic, onion powder, white pepper, oregano, and thyme.
2. **Place** fish in an ungreased 13″ x 9″ x 2″ baking pan.
3. **Sprinkle** lemon juice and seasoning mixture evenly over fish.
4. **Drizzle** melted margarine or butter evenly over fish portions.
5. **Bake** for 20-25 minutes until fish **flakes** easily with a fork.

Nutrients per serving
2.5 ounce portion, cooked

Calories	149	Saturated Fat	1.4 g	Iron	.4 mg
Protein	17 g	Cholesterol	54 mg	Calcium	26 mg
Carbohydrate	1 g	Vitamin A	71 RE	Sodium	80 mg
Total Fat	8.2 g	Vitamin C	1 mg	Dietary Fiber	0 g

HOW TO EAT TO FEEL GOOD

Young children can't always eat full size meals. So when choosing snack foods — keep your eye on your main goal — a balanced diet. Snack on whole wheat toast, breadsticks, cheese cubes, hard-boiled eggs, cut up fruits, raw veggie sticks and lowfat dip (See pg 17). Try a variety of lowfat and nonfat yogurts.

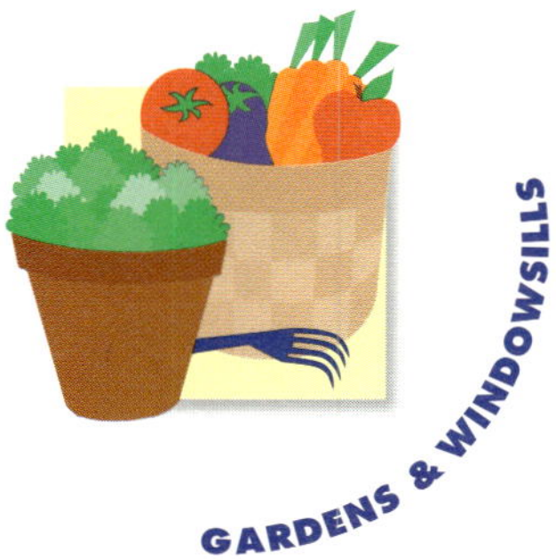

This winter, take your child to a public library. Take out a book about kids and gardening. Look for seed catalogues. Start planning your indoor or outdoor garden — for the spring.

School Lunch Recipe

Vegetable Chili

30 minutes Serves: 5

- **1** Tbsp vegetable oil
- ¼ cup fresh green peppers, diced
- ½ cup onions, diced
- **1** Tbsp chili powder
- **2** tsp cumin
- ½ tsp granulated garlic
- ¼ tsp onion powder
- **1½** tsp red hot sauce (optional)
- **1** Tbsp brown sugar, firmly packed
- **1½** cups canned crushed tomatoes
- ¼ cup canned diced tomatoes, drained
- **2** cup canned kidney beans, drained, rinsed
- ¼ cup *plus* 2 Tbsp bulgur wheat, (No. 3 size)
- **1** cup water
- ½ cup lowfat plain yogurt
- ½ cup *plus* 2 Tbsp lowfat cheddar cheese, shredded

1. In a large sauce pan, **heat** oil over medium heat until hot.
2. **Add** peppers and **saute** over medium heat for 3 minutes until tender.
3. **Add** onions and **saute** for 2 minutes until translucent.
4. In a small bowl, **combine** chili powder, cumin, garlic, onion powder, red hot sauce (optional), brown sugar, crushed tomato, and diced tomatoes.
5. **Add** tomato mixture to cooked vegetables and **simmer**, uncovered, for 10 minutes.
6. **Mix** in kidney beans, bulgur wheat, and water. **Simmer**, uncovered, for 15 minutes.
7. **Blend** in yogurt and **stir** to blend.
8. **Sprinkle** 2 Tbsp of cheddar cheese over each serving.

Nutrients per serving
1 cup

Calories	215	Saturated Fat	0.8 g	Iron	2.7 mg
Protein	10 g	Cholesterol	1 mg	Calcium	104 mg
Carbohydrate	37 g	Vitamin A	118 RE	Sodium	636 mg
Total Fat	4.1 g	Vitamin C	24 mg	Dietary Fiber	7 g

Oranges in Tangerine Juice

10 minutes Serves: 1

Try this in the morning before your child goes to school. It makes a nice lunchtime snack.

1 orange
Juice of **1** tangerine

1. With a sharp paring knife, **slice** the top and bottom part of the orange off, so that the orange can sit flat on either end. **Carve** the remaining orange skin off, starting at the top of the orange, carving your way down around the shape of the orange, eliminating the skin and white pithy part, exposing just the fruit.
2. When all the skin is removed, **cut** the orange into sections by making incisions at each section of the orange, letting them drop into a small bowl. **Squeeze** the remaining orange juice over the orange sections.
3. **Squeeze** the tangerine, and pour juice over the orange pieces.

Nutrients per serving
1 orange and juice

Calories	100	Saturated Fat	0 g	Iron	.3 mg
Protein	2 g	Cholesterol	0 mg	Calcium	61 mg
Carbohydrate	24 g	Vitamin A	44 RE	Sodium	0 mg
Total Fat	.3 g	Vitamin C	113 mg	Dietary Fiber	3 g

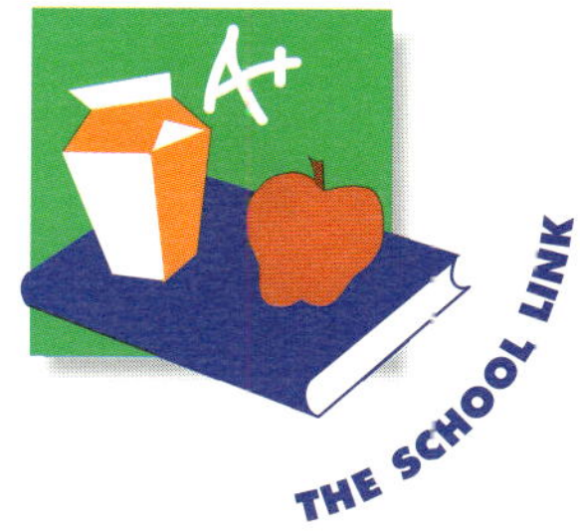

Make a healthy snack after school at home. Try "winter reindeer." Spread peanut butter on whole wheat bread triangles. Make eyes and nose with raisins. Use twisted pretzels as antlers. Enjoy.

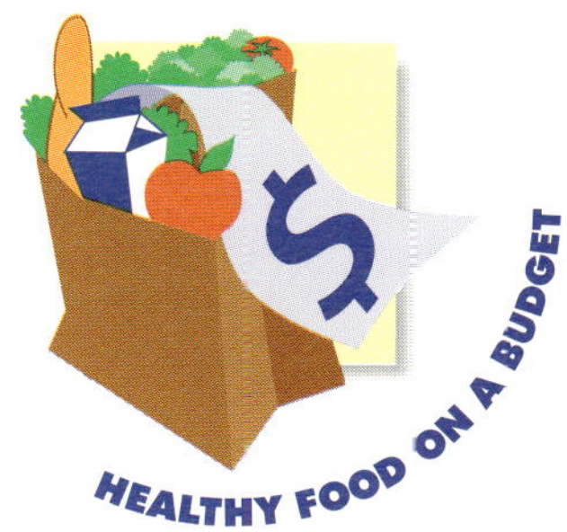

Instead of store-bought snacks, make your own cereal mix, granola mix, different flavored popcorns, pretzels and cut-up vegetables at home.

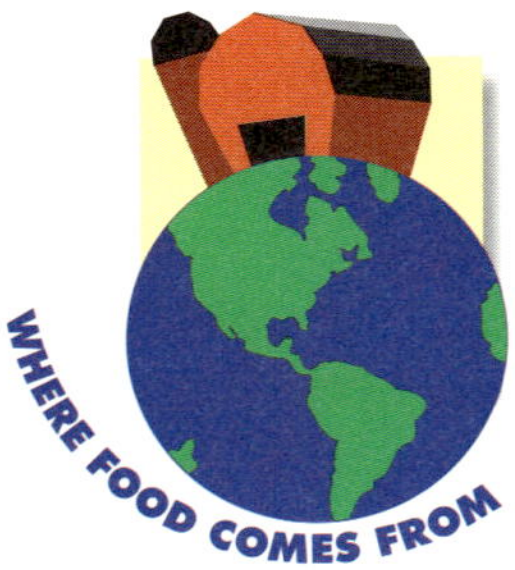

Introduce your child to different forms a food can take. At snacktime, let your child choose raw apple, apple juice, or applesauce — or a small amount of all three. Talk about different textures of these foods, which one your child likes best, and why.

Carrot Bars

25–30 minutes Serves: 40 pieces

You can make this recipe with a similar amount of cooked pumpkin, cooked sweet potato or banana.

- **1** cup sugar
- **½** cup vegetable oil
- **¼** cup applesauce
- **2** jars baby food carrots
- **2** eggs, beaten
- **1¼** cup flour
- **1** tsp vanilla
- **1** tsp baking soda
- **1** tsp cinnamon
- **½** tsp salt
- **½** cup nuts, chopped (optional)

Icing (optional)

- **¼** cup soft margarine
- **1½** cups powdered sugar
- **3** oz light cream cheese
- **1** tsp vanilla

Preheat oven to 350° degrees F.

1. In a large bowl, **mix** sugar, oil, applesauce, baby food carrots, eggs, flour, 1 tsp of vanilla, baking soda, cinnamon, salt and nuts (optional) together.
2. **Bake** in 13″ x 9″ greased and floured pan for 25–30 minutes.
3. While bars **bake, mix** icing (optional): margarine, powdered sugar, light cream cheese, and 1 tsp vanilla.
3. When bars are baked, **cool, spread** with icing or sprinkle with powdered sugar. Cut into bars. Serve.

Nutrients per serving
1 piece

Calories	71	Saturated Fat	0.5 g	Iron	0.3 mg
Protein	1 g	Cholesterol	11 mg	Calcium	4 mg
Carbohydrate	10 g	Vitamin A	86 RE	Sodium	73 mg
Total Fat	3 g	Vitamin C	0 mg	Dietary Fiber	0 g

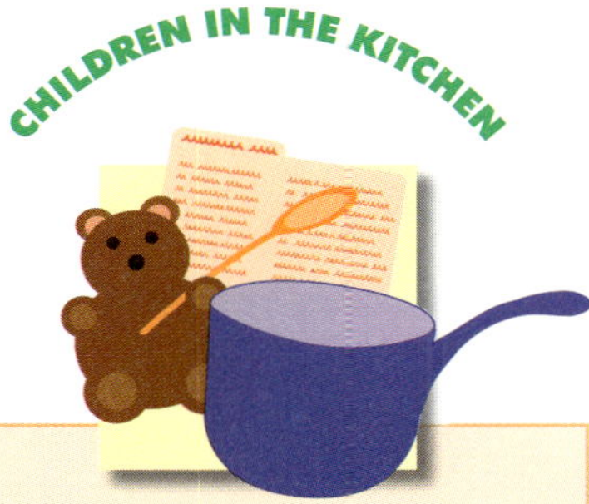

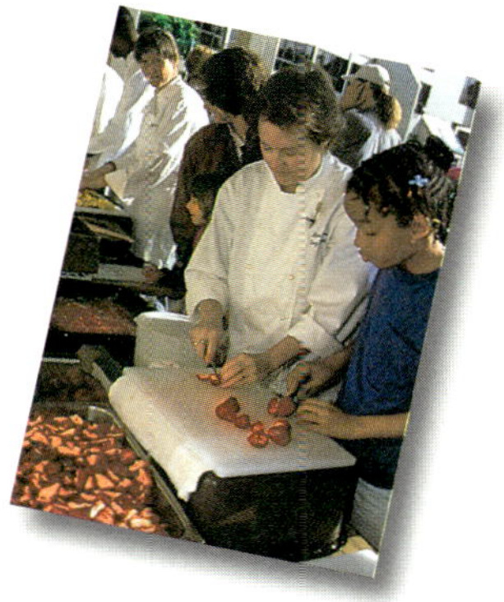

Knothole Egg

5 minutes Serves: 4

You can make this one at a time, two at a time, or four at a time. To make all four at once, you'll need a 4-piece toaster and a large skillet. If you don't have a large toaster, make one or two, and repeat. Try rye, whole wheat or pumpernickle bread.

4 slices of bread
4 eggs
4 Tbsp butter or soft margarine

1. **Toast** the four slices of bread in a toaster. Show children how to **cut** a hole in the center of each slice of toast, using two-inch cookie cutters or small empty juice glasses.
2. Supervise the children while they **crack** one egg each into four cups. Be careful not to break the yolk!
3. **Melt** the butter or margarine over medium-low heat. When it has melted, **lift** the skillet and **tilt** it to evenly **coat** the pan. Direct children to **put** the toast in the pan, and **pour** one egg into each hole in the center of each piece of toast. The white will run over the edge of the toast, but that's okay. **Turn** the heat as low as possible. **Grill** until lightly brown.
4. **Turn** each piece of bread-with-an-egg-in-the-middle over, and let it lightly brown. Slide onto serving plates. Eat at once!

Nutrients per serving
1 egg with bread

Calories	158	Saturated Fat	2.1 g	Iron	1.5 mg
Protein	8 g	Cholesterol	211 mg	Calcium	52 mg
Carbohydrate	13 g	Vitamin A	114 RE	Sodium	298 mg
Total Fat	7.8 g	Vitamin C	0 mg	Dietary Fiber	1 g

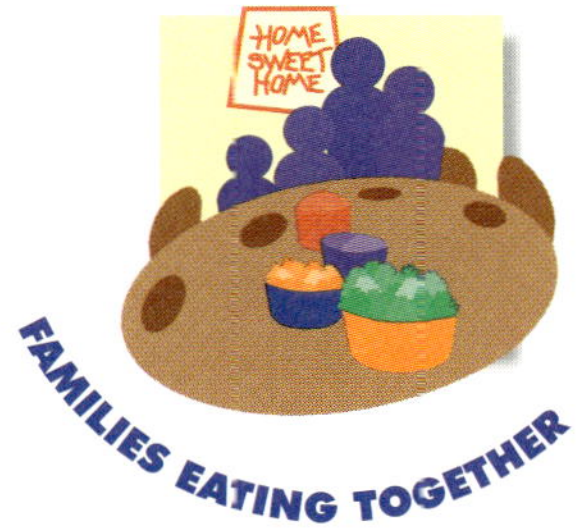

Have a family snacking party. Ask each family member to make a healthy snack; sample each snack and discuss what you liked and didn't like, and why.

HOW TO EAT TO FEEL GOOD

Breads, cereals, rice and pasta are the foundation for a healthful diet. Some people think starchy foods like bread, noodles and rice are fattening. But really, it's the fats, oils and sweets you add to these foods that increase the calories. Eating plenty of plain, starchy foods is a good way to fill up with fewer calories.

School Lunch Recipe

Vegetable Lasagna

1 hour Serves: 12

Try a vegetarian entree for a change.

- **1** lb lasagna noodles (18 each)
- **1** Tbsp vegetable oil
- **¾** cup fresh zucchini, sliced
- **½** cup fresh mushrooms, sliced
- **⅓** cup onions, diced
- **1** Tbsp *plus* 1 tsp all-purpose flour

- **2** cups frozen broccoli pieces

- **3** cups tomato sauce
- **¾** cup tomato paste
- **1** Tbsp *plus* 1 tsp oregano leaves
- **½** tsp garlic powder

- **3¼** cups lowfat cottage cheese, drained
- **1** Tbsp parsley flakes
- **½** tsp garlic powder
- **¼** cup *plus* **2** Tbsp dry bread crumbs

- **2** Tbsp grated parmesan cheese
- **1½** cups lowfat mozzarella cheese, shredded

- **¼** cup grated parmesan cheese (optional)

Preheat oven to 375°.

Noodles:

1. In a large sauce pan, **cook** noodles in boiling water for 10-12 minutes until firm-tender. **Drain** and **hold** in cold water.
2. In a medium skillet, **heat** vegetable oil over medium heat until hot. **Add** the zucchini, mushrooms, and onions and **saute** for 3 minutes until tender. **Stir** in flour and **cook** for 3 minutes. Do not brown. **Remove** from heat and **set aside.**
3. **Add** broccoli to boiling water and **cook** for 3 minutes until tender. **Drain** and **rinse** broccoli in cold water.

Sauce:

4. In a medium sauce pan, **combine** tomato sauce, tomato paste, oregano, and garlic powder. **Simmer,** uncovered, over low heat for 20 minutes.
5. **Add** sauteed vegetables and cooked broccoli to sauce and **stir** to combine. **Simmer,** uncovered, for 10 minutes.

(continued on back of card)

Vegetable Lasagna, continued

Cheese mix:

6. In a medium mixing bowl, **combine** cottage cheese, parsley, garlic powder, and bread crumbs. **Stir** well to blend.

   In a small bowl, **combine** 2 Tbsp parmesan cheese and mozzarella cheese.

   Spread ½ cup of vegetable sauce evenly in a lightly greased 13″ x 9″ x 2″ baking pan.

Assembly:

First layer —

6 lasagna noodles

half of cottage cheese mixture

1¼ cups vegetable sauce

half of parmesan-mozzarella cheese mixture

Second layer —

Repeat first layer, **using** remainder of cottage cheese mixture and parmesan-mozzarella mixture.

Third layer —

Top with 6 lasagna noodles and remainder of vegetable sauce

Sprinkle the rest of parmesan cheese (optional) over assembled lasagna. **Cover** with foil. **Bake** for 60 minutes until bubbling.

Remove from oven and allow lasagna **to sit** for 15 minutes before serving. **Cut** lasagna into 12 pieces (3 x 4).

Nutrients per serving
1 piece

Calories	297	Saturated Fat	1.9 g	Iron	3.3 mg
Protein	20 g	Cholesterol	8 mg	Calcium	201 mg
Carbohydrate	45 g	Vitamin A	162 RE	Sodium	747 mg
Total Fat	4.8 g	Vitamin C	24 mg	Dietary Fiber	4 g

THE SCHOOL LINK

Ask your children to count how many servings of grain products they had today at school lunch and as a snack (3-4 small crackers count in this group as a serving). And a tortilla is one serving!

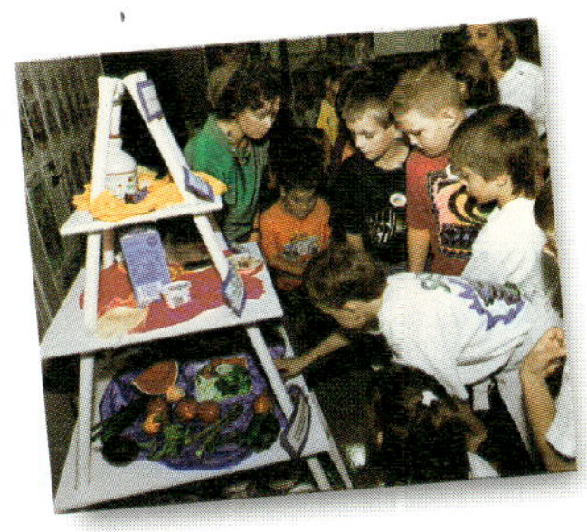

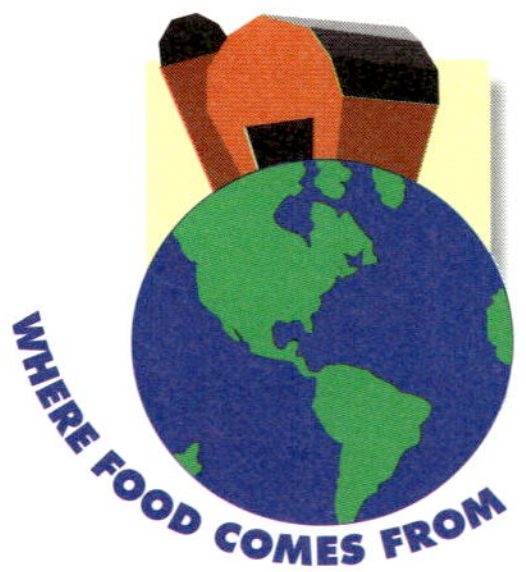

Show your kids bread doesn't come from a bag. Visit a bakery. Or bake muffins or bread at home with your kids.

School Lunch Recipe

Tabouleh (tah-BUHL-lee)

30 minutes Serves: 13

Here's a popular Middle Eastern dish that adds fiber to your diet!

- **1½** cups bulgur wheat (No. 3 size)
- **1½** cups boiling water
- **3** cups fresh tomatoes, diced
- **1½** cups fresh cucumber, peeled, seeded, diced
- **¼** cups fresh parsley, chopped
- **¼** cup *plus* 2 Tbsp onions, minced
- **2** tsp fresh mint, chopped, or ¼ tsp dried
- **¼** tsp cumin (optional)
- **1** tsp salt
- **¼** cup lemon juice
- **2** Tbsp vegetable oil

1. **Combine** bulgur and boiling water. **Let stand** for 30 minutes or until water is absorbed. Do not drain.
2. **Add** tomatoes, cucumbers, parsley, onions, mint, and cumin (optional) to the bulgur and **stir** to blend.
3. In a small bowl, **combine** salt and lemon juice. Slowly **whisk** in oil.
4. **Add** dressing to salad and **toss** to coat all ingredients. Serve chilled.

Nutrients per serving
½ cup

Calories	91	Saturated Fat	.4 g	Iron	.7 mg
Protein	3 g	Cholesterol	0 mg	Calcium	15 mg
Carbohydrate	16 g	Vitamin A	29 RE	Sodium	188 mg
Total Fat	2.5 g	Vitamin C	11 mg	Dietary Fiber	4 g

Sweet Potatoes with Lime

45 to 60 minutes Serves: 8

To save time: Bake sweet potatoes in a microwave oven.

4 sweet potatoes, washed and pricked
juice of 2 limes
3-4 cilantro leaves (optional)
¼ tsp salt (optional)

Preheat oven to 375°F

1. **Bake** the sweet potatoes whole in their skins, until tender, about 45 minutes to 1 hour.
2. When the potatoes are tender, **slit** open the skin, and **scoop** out the flesh onto a serving dish. **Season** with salt (optional).
3. **Squeeze** fresh lime juice over the top, and **sprinkle** with 3 or 4 cilantro leaves (optional).

Nutrients per serving
½ cup

Calories	61	Saturated Fat	0 g	Iron	.3 mg
Protein	1 g	Cholesterol	0 mg	Calcium	16 mg
Carbohydrate	15 g	Vitamin A	1243 RE	Sodium	5 mg
Total Fat	.1 g	Vitamin C	17 mg	Dietary Fiber	2 g

HEALTHY FOOD ON A BUDGET

Put breads, pasta and rice in the center of your menus. They cost less than many other foods. Use beans and small amounts of meat and cheese together with pasta, rice or other grains to make lower cost main dishes.

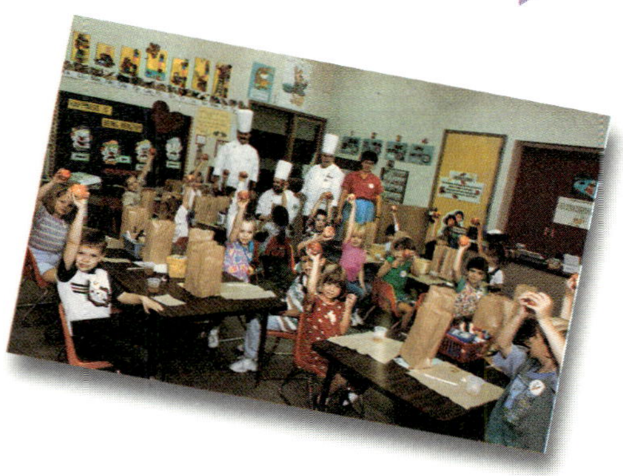

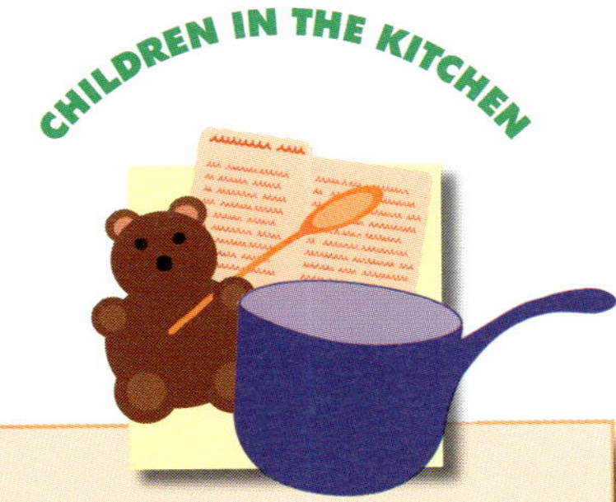

School Lunch Recipe

New Oatmeal Raisin Cookies

10–13 minutes Serves: 2½ dozen cookies

- ¾ cup sugar
- **2** Tbsp margarine or butter
- **1** fresh large egg
- **2** Tbsp lowfat milk
- ¼ cup canned applesauce
- ¾ cup all-purpose flour
- ¼ tsp baking soda
- ½ tsp ground cinnamon
- ⅛ tsp ground nutmeg
- ¼ tsp salt
- 1¼ cup quick oats
- ½ cup raisins

Preheat oven to 350°F.

1. Guide children in using an electric mixer on medium speed, **Cream** sugar and margarine or butter until smooth and creamy.
2. Ask child to slowly **add** egg. **Mix** on medium speed for 1 minute.
3. Child can slowly **add** milk and applesauce. **Mix** for 1 more minute. **Scrape** the sides of the bowl.
4. In a small bowl, help child **combine** together flour, baking soda, cinnamon, nutmeg, and salt. **Add** dry ingredients gradually to the creamed mixture and **mix** on low speed for 2 minutes, until blended.
5. **Add** oats and raisins and **blend** for 30 seconds on low speed. **Scrape** the sides of the bowl.
6. Child can **portion** dough by rounded teaspoons onto lightly greased cookie sheets.

   Bake for 10-13 minutes until lightly browned. **Cool** on a wire rack. Yummy!

Nutrients per serving
1 cookie

Calories	70	Saturated Fat	.3 g	Iron	.4 mg
Protein	1 g	Cholesterol	8 mg	Calcium	7 mg
Carbohydrate	14 g	Vitamin A	14 RE	Sodium	42 mg
Total Fat	1.3 g	Vitamin C	0 mg	Dietary Fiber	1 g

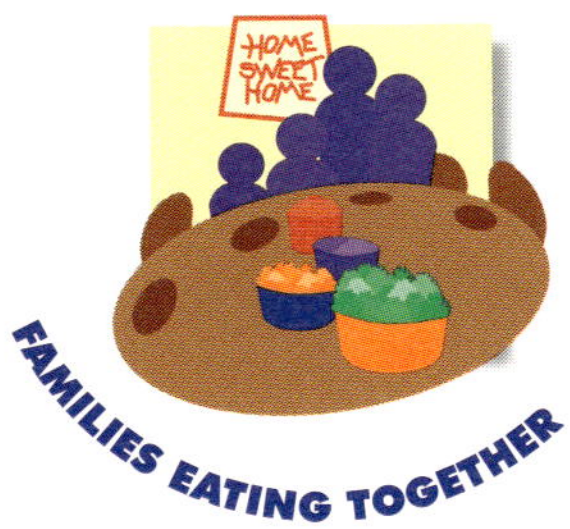

Hot cereal is a nutritious breakfast that the family can make together: oatmeal, grits or cream of wheat. Try using fruit such as applesauce or peaches as a topping instead of sugar.

Taco Pie

School Lunch Recipe

30 minutes Serves: 12

- **1** lb 8 oz lean ground beef, no more than 24% fat
- **¼** cup taco seasoning mix
- **½** cup water
- **½** cup *plus* 2 Tbsp salsa
- **½** cup *plus* 2 Tbsp tomato paste
- **½** cup *plus* 2 Tbsp water
- **1½** Tbsp taco seasoning mix
- **7** flour tortillas, 8″
- **2** cups lowfat cheddar cheese, shredded

Preheat oven to 350°F.

1. In a large skillet, **brown** ground beef until no signs of pink remain.
2. **Drain** fat from beef and **discard**. **Return** beef to stovetop.
3. **Add** ¼ cup taco seasoning mix and ½ cup water to cooked beef and **stir** to combine. **Simmer** for 15 minutes.
4. In a bowl, **combine** salsa, tomato paste, water and taco seasoning mix.
5. **Cut** tortillas in halves (14 half-tortillas) and assemble:

Bottom Layer:
In a lightly greased 13″ x 9″ x 2″ baking pan, **lay** 5 half-tortillas.

Spread ½ cup of the salsa mixture on top of the tortillas. **Distribute** 1½ cups of the cooked meat mixture evenly over the salsa. **Top** with ½ cup of shredded cheese.

(continued on back of card)

HOW TO EAT TO FEEL GOOD

Balance is the key to choosing a lower fat diet. You don't have to give up all high fat foods. It's your average intake over a few days, not a single food or even a single meal that's important. Learn which foods are high in fat and which are low in fat. Eat fewer high fat food choices or eat them less often.

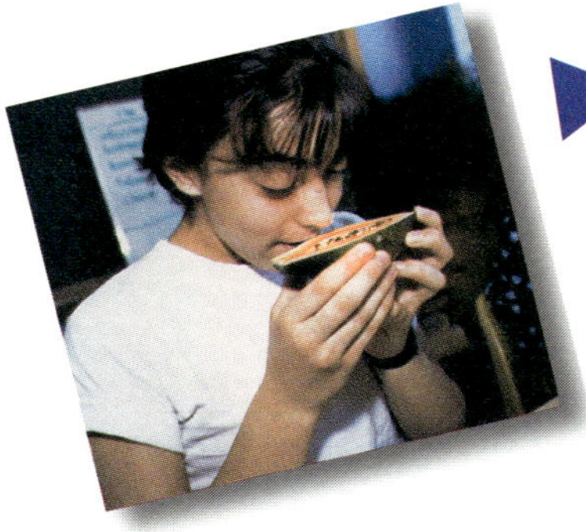

THE SCHOOL LINK

How can your children reduce fat at lunch meals? Talk about choosing mustard instead of mayonnaise on sandwiches and lower fat dressings at salad bars. Team Nutrition schools are now serving lower fat food choices! Encourage your child to choose them.

Taco Pie, continued

Middle Layer:
Lay 4 half-tortillas on top of the cheese. **Repeat as for first layer, using** the remainder of the, salsa meat mixture, and cheese.

Top Layer:
Lay 5 half-tortillas on top of the cheese. **Spread** the remainder of the salsa mixture on top of the tortillas and **sprinkle** remainder of cheese evenly over top.

6. **Cover** with foil. **Bake** for 30 minutes or until thoroughly heated.

   Allow pie to **rest** for 5 minutes before portioning. **Cut** pie into 12 pieces.

Nutrients per serving
1 piece

Calories	268	Saturated Fat	4.0 g	Iron	3.3 mg
Protein	20 g	Cholesterol	44 mg	Calcium	141 mg
Carbohydrate	22 g	Vitamin A	114 RE	Sodium	345 mg
Total Fat	11.2 g	Vitamin C	7 mg	Dietary Fiber	2 g

School Lunch Recipe

Hearty Vegetable Soup

35 minutes Serves: 6

- *1 cup water
- *1½ Tbsp dry pinto beans
- 1½ cups water
- 1 qt vegetable or chicken broth
- 2 Tbsp dry lentils
- ¼ cup pearled barley
- ¼ cup onions, diced
- ½ cup fresh carrots, diced
- ¼ cup fresh celery, diced
- ½ cup fresh white potatoes, peeled, cubed
- 1 Tbsp tomato paste
- ½ tsp white pepper
- ½ cup frozen corn
- ½ cup frozen cut green beans
- ½ cup fresh cabbage, shredded (optional)

1. ***SOAK BEANS:**
   Overnight Method: **Add** 1 cup of cold water to dry pinto beans. **Cover** and let stand in a refrigerator overnight. **Discard** the water and **rinse** beans.
   Quick-soak method: **Bring** 1 cup of water to a boil. **Add** dry pinto beans and **boil** for 2 minutes. **Remove** from heat and **allow to soak** for 1 hour. **Discard** the water and **rinse** beans.
2. In a large saucepan, bring 1½ cups water and vegetable or chicken broth to a boil.
3. **Add** soaked pinto beans, lentils, barley, onions, carrots, celery, potatoes, tomato paste, and white pepper. **Cover** and **simmer** for 20 minutes.
4. **Add** corn, green beans, and cabbage (optional) and **simmer**, covered, for 15 minutes.

Nutrients per serving
1 cup

Calories	122	Saturated Fat	.3 g	Iron	1.7 mg
Protein	8 g	Cholesterol	0 mg	Calcium	31 mg
Carbohydrate	21 g	Vitamin A	321 RE	Sodium	65 mg
Total Fat	1.4 g	Vitamin C	8 mg	Dietary Fiber	5 g

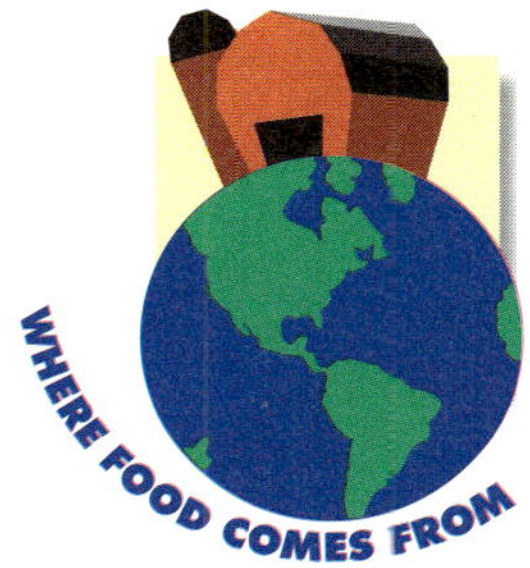

Fats, oils and sweets are often hidden in foods. Check the number of grams of fat on food labels. Look in your cupboards and compare labels.

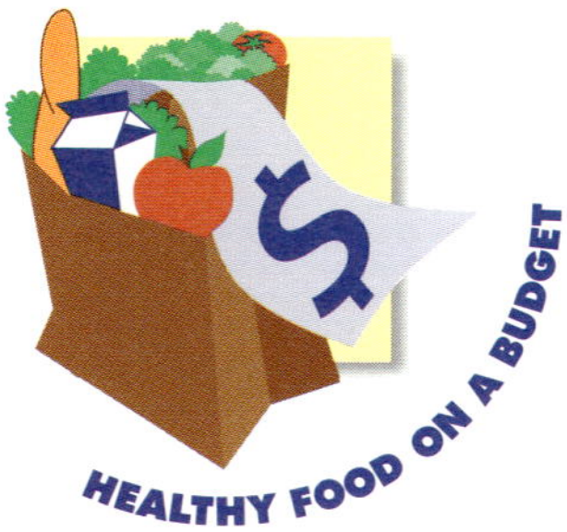

Some new lowfat packaged foods may cost more than their regular counterparts. Take a look at labels and compare products for price, fat and calories before you buy.

School Lunch Recipe

Whole Wheat Sugar Cookies

10–13 minutes Serves: 2½ dozen cookies

- ¼ cup *plus* 2 Tbsp margarine or butter
- ¾ cup sugar
- **1** fresh large egg
- ¾ tsp vanilla
- **2** Tbsp lowfat milk
- 1½ cups whole wheat flour
- ¾ tsp baking powder
- ½ tsp baking soda
- ½ tsp salt
- ⅛ tsp ground nutmeg
- ½ tsp ground cinnamon

Sprinkle:

- **2** Tbsp sugar
- **1** tsp ground cinnamon

Preheat oven to 375°F.

1. Using an electric mixer on medium speed, **cream** margarine or butter and ¾ cup sugar until light and fluffy.
2. **Add** egg, vanilla, and milk and **mix** for one minute until smooth. **Scrape** the sides of the bowl.
3. In a small bowl, **combine** together flour, baking powder, baking soda, salt, nutmeg, and cinnamon. **Add** dry ingredients gradually to the creamed mixture and **mix** on low speed for one minute until well blended. **Scrape** the sides of the bowl.
4. **Portion** dough by rounded teaspoons onto lightly greased cookie sheets.
5. **Combine** 2 Tbsp sugar and 1 tsp cinnamon and **sprinkle** over cookies.
6. **Bake** for 10-13 minutes, until lightly browned. **Cool** on wire rack.

Nutrients per serving
1 cookie

Calories	76	Saturated Fat	.6 g	Iron	.4 mg
Protein	1 g	Cholesterol	8 mg	Calcium	14 mg
Carbohydrate	12 g	Vitamin A	32 RE	Sodium	102 mg
Total Fat	2.6 g	Vitamin C	0 mg	Dietary Fiber	1 g

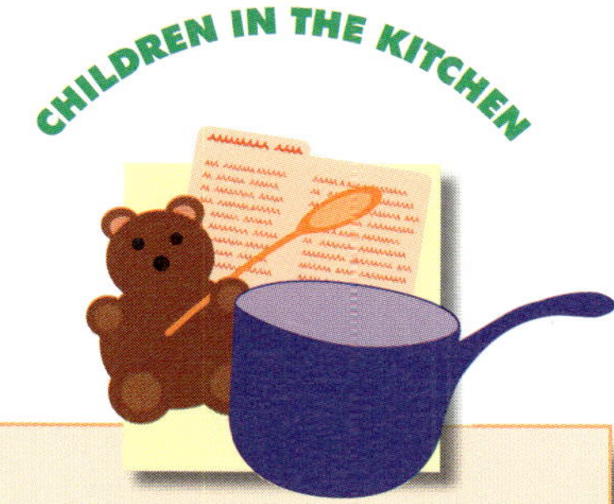

Granola-Topped French Toast (Overnight)

30 minutes Serves: 8–10

For overnight slumber parties, get kids to help "prepare" their breakfast the night before.

- **1** large loaf (1 pound) of French bread, cut into 1-inch cubes
- **4** eggs
- **3** cups skim milk or 1% lowfat
- **1** tsp vanilla extract
- **½** tsp ground cinnamon
- **½** cup raisins (or dried cranberries)

Topping

- **3** Tbsp margarine
- **2** Tbsp honey or maple syrup
- **1** cup brown sugar
- **½** cup lowfat granola or chopped walnuts

The night before:

1. Children can **spray** a 9″ x 13″ baking dish and scoop in the cubed bread; spread into an even layer.
2. Children can help **break** the eggs into a large bowl and **beat** them lightly. Children can **add** milk, vanilla, cinnamon and raisins (or cranberries) and **mix** thoroughly.
3. Children can **pour** the milk and egg mixture over the bread, making certain all the bread is softened. **Cover** tightly with plastic wrap and **refrigerate** overnight.

For breakfast: Preheat oven to 350°F.
In a small pan, **melt** the margarine, honey or syrup, and brown sugar. **Mix** in the granola or nuts. **Drop** by spoonfuls over the top of the bread and bake for 30 minutes.

Remove from oven and cool several minutes. Let children serve themselves.

Nutrients per serving
1 serving

Calories	342	Saturated Fat	2 g	Iron	2.2 mg
Protein	10 g	Cholesterol	91 mg	Calcium	165 mg
Carbohydrate	57 g	Vitamin A	137 RE	Sodium	438 mg
Total Fat	8.5 g	Vitamin C	1 mg	Dietary Fiber	2 g

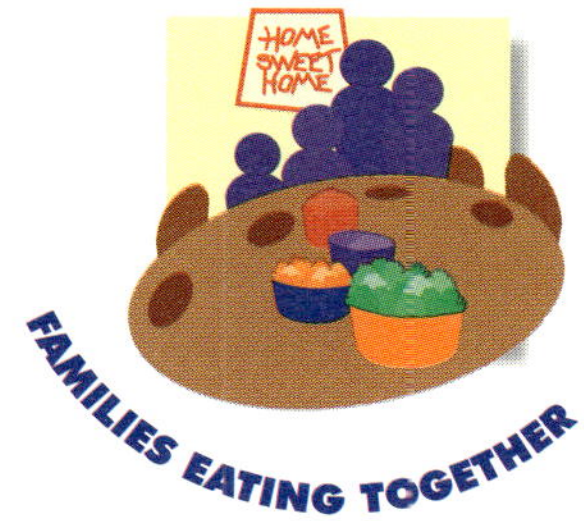

Celebrate Valentine's Day with a lower fat version of your favorite cake. See how to modify your home recipes on pg 83.

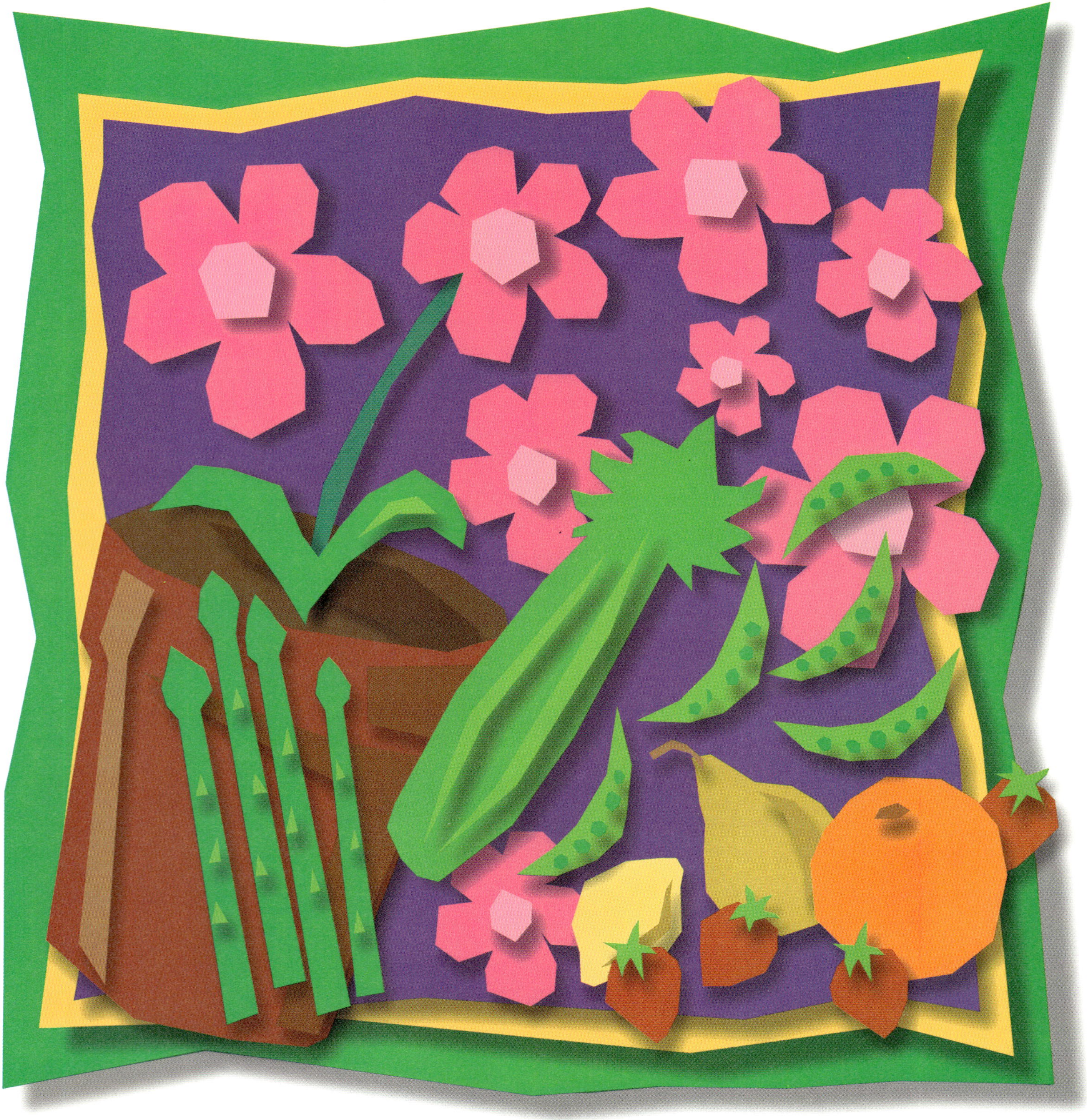

Spring

Spring is the season of renewal. New crops push up above the ground, and animals give birth. Winter's ice thaws, rains come; the earth smells fresh. In the markets, a few new vegetables and fruits show up.

Spring Chef Teams Included:

Susan Feniger, Mary Sue Milliken, Nancy Silverton, Evan Kleiman, Andrea Crawford, Tommy Tang, Michael Lomonaco, Anne Rosenzweig, Douglas Rodrigues, Alexander Small, Jimmy Schmidt, Lorraine Platman, Odessa Piper, Peter Loren, Harlan "Pete" Peterson and Brian Polcyn.

In most parts of the country, however, the coming of spring doesn't bring the full seasonal bounty that occurs later, in the summer and fall. Still, there are nice, seasonal bargains. As always, foods from the foundation of the Food Guide Pyramid, the Bread, Cereal, Rice and Pasta Group, are readily available. Nor are foods from the Milk, Yogurt and Cheese Group seasonal. These are as important as ever, rich in protein and calcium; the best choices for those age 2 and over are the lowfat varieties. If you drink whole milk, consider switching to 2%, or

1%, or skim milk, which has all the protein and calcium and other nutrients, but less fat.

The Meat, Poultry, Fish, Dry Beans, Eggs and Nuts groups are also widely available. Spring is the season of "spring chickens," which are younger and more tender. Spring runs of fish, such as smelt and salmon, can be delicious. Beef, lamb and pork are always available.

In the Fruit Group, apples are still available, as are citrus fruits, and we begin to see, later in the season, strawberries. In the Vegetable group, asparagus is always a sign of spring. Artichokes begin to come in, as do peas. Spinach is available. Lettuces start to be more affordable. Celery comes in. Scallions, or green onions, are in season. At the same time, hardier vegetables, such as potatoes and sweet potatoes, winter squash, cauliflower, carrots and cabbage, and many kinds of dark greens are still inexpensive. For a quick and tasty way to cook greens, see Seared Greens pg 54. For use of a variety of vegetables, try Early Vegetable and Lentil Salad, pg 55. Summer is not far away!

In Season:

Vegetables:
Artichokes, asparagus, beets, broccoli, cabbage, carrots, cauliflower, celery, lettuce, onions, peas, potatoes, spinach.

Fruits:
Apples, avocados, grapefruit, lemons, navel oranges, Valencia oranges, strawberries, pears.

Also,
All dairy, meats and poultry products, most fish and shellfish.

Chicken Salad Roll Ups

20 minutes Serves: 6

This rolled-up sandwich might be the perfect answer to the leftover chicken dilemma. You can use any leftover poultry, such as turkey.

6 flour tortillas, 7" in diameter

Vinaigrette

- **1½** Tbsp olive oil
- **1½** Tbsp vinegar
- **1** Tbsp grainy mustard
- **½** Tbsp coarsely ground black pepper

Chicken Salad Filling

- **3½** cups cooked, shredded chicken, loosely packed
- **12** large Chinese cabbage leaves, shredded
- **1** medium sweet red pepper, cut into very thin strips
- **8** green onions, sliced
- **4** celery stalks, sliced
- **1** package (about 6 ounces) alfalfa sprouts

1. In a large bowl, **combine** all the ingredients for the filling except for the sprouts. **Pour** the vinaigrette over, **toss** until blended. **Set** aside.
2. **Place** ⅙ of the chicken salad filling in a line along one side of each tortilla. **Add** sprouts as desired and **roll up** like an enchilada.
3. **Serve** immediately. Or, finished sandwiches can be **wrapped** individually in plastic and **stored** for up to 24 hours. **Cut** each roll in half diagonally, and **place** on the serving plate in a "**V**" shape with the cut ends facing up.

Nutrients per serving
1 rollup

Calories	330	Saturated Fat	2.6 g	Iron	3.3 mg
Protein	29 g	Cholesterol	72 mg	Calcium	126 mg
Carbohydrate	26 g	Vitamin A	226 RE	Sodium	317 mg
Total Fat	12.4 g	Vitamin C	58 mg	Dietary Fiber	4 g

HOW TO EAT TO FEEL GOOD

The new Nutrition Facts label makes it easier to know what is in the food you eat. One way to use the label is to look for nutrient content claims such as "free," "low" or "reduced" on the front of the label to identify foods low in calories, fat, cholesterol and sodium. Compare labels on two similar foods to make an informed choice.

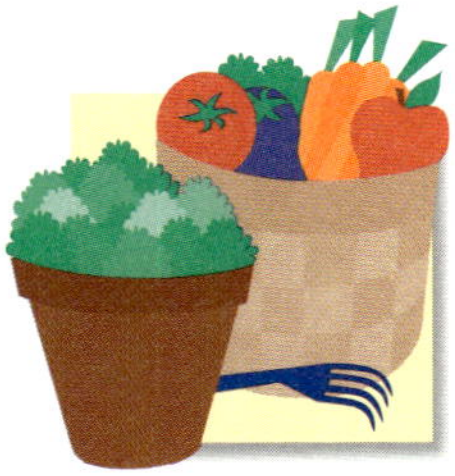

GARDENS & WINDOWSILLS

Now in springtime you can start planting the garden. Plant a "theme garden," such as a salad or herb garden or a garden to supply pizza toppings. Include a small child's garden. For a preschooler, a two-foot plot is fine. The adult should prepare the soil — it's hard work for kids. Make rows small.

School Lunch Recipe

Breakfast Burrito with Salsa

30 minutes Serves: 4

- **4** fresh large eggs
- **2** Tbsp frozen corn
- **1** Tbsp lowfat milk
- **2** Tbsp fresh green peppers, diced
- ¼ cup onions, minced
- **1** Tbsp fresh tomatoes, diced
- **1** tsp prepared mustard
- ¼ tsp granulated garlic
- ¼ tsp hot pepper sauce (optional)
- **4** flour tortillas, 8-inch
- ½ cup canned salsa

Preheat oven to 350°F.

1. In a large mixing bowl, **blend** the eggs, corn, milk, green peppers, onions, tomatoes, mustard, garlic, hot pepper sauce, and salt for 1 minute until eggs are smooth.
2. **Pour** egg mixture into a lightly oiled 9" x 9" x 2" baking dish and **cover** with foil.
3. **Bake** for 20-25 minutes until eggs are set and thoroughly cooked.
4. **Wrap** tortillas in plastic and **microwave** for 20 seconds until warm. Be careful when unwrapping the tortillas. The steam can be hot
5. **Cut** baked egg mixture into 4 equal pieces and **roll** 1 piece of cooked egg in each tortilla.
6. **Serve** each burrito topped with 2 Tbsp of salsa.

Nutrients per serving
1 burrito

Calories	208	Saturated Fat	2.0 g	Iron	2.2 mg
Protein	10 g	Cholesterol	212 mg	Calcium	61 mg
Carbohydrate	24 g	Vitamin A	124 RE	Sodium	331 mg
Total Fat	8 g	Vitamin C	12 mg	Dietary Fiber	2 g

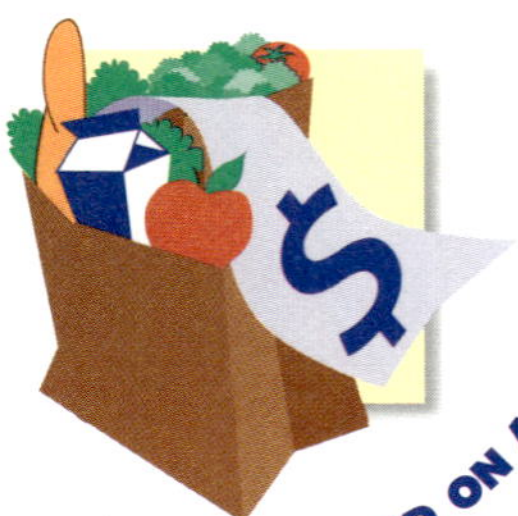

HEALTHY FOOD ON A BUDGET

Many stores provide unit price labels to help customers make informed price decisions. Look for shelf labeling to help you compare the price of similar products.

School Lunch Recipe

Marinated Black Bean Salad

30 minutes to marinate Serves: 10

- **2¼** cups canned black beans, drained, rinsed
- **2** cups frozen corn
- **½** cup fresh green pepper, minced
- **½** cup fresh red pepper, minced
- **¼** cup onions, minced
- **1½** tsp lemon juice
- **1** tsp parsley flakes
- **⅛** tsp ground cumin
- **⅛** tsp garlic powder
- **1** cup salsa
- **1** tsp vegetable oil
- **¾** cup Monterey Jack cheese, shredded (optional)

1. In a bowl, **combine** black beans, corn, peppers, and onions.
2. In a small bowl, **whisk** together lemon juice, parsley, cumin, garlic powder, salsa, and oil.
3. **Pour** dressing over vegetables and **stir** to coat.
4. **Cover** and **refrigerate** for at least 30 minutes or longer to marinate.
5. Before serving, **sprinkle** Monterey Jack cheese (optional) over top of salad.

Nutrients per serving
½ cup

Calories	133	Saturated Fat	.2 g	Iron	1.3 mg
Protein	4 g	Cholesterol	0 mg	Calcium	35 mg
Carbohydrate	15 g	Vitamin A	74 RE	Sodium	220 mg
Total Fat	.9 g	Vitamin C	31 mg	Dietary Fiber	3 g

THE SCHOOL LINK

March is National Nutrition Month. Ask your children to make a Nutrition Facts Label poster to hang on the cafeteria wall. They can present this poster to the food service staff. Ask the staff for the nutrition information for a day's menu.

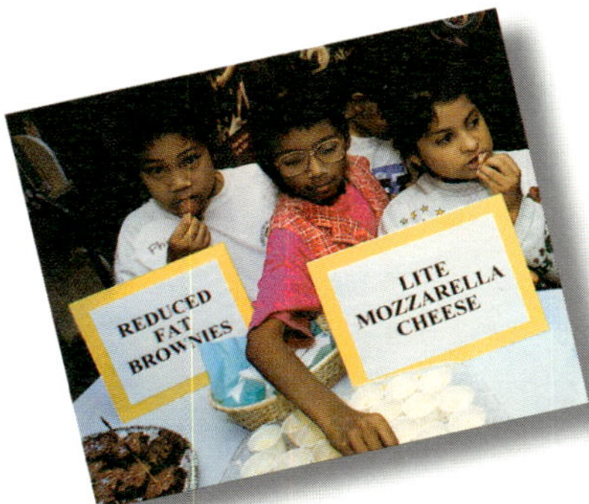

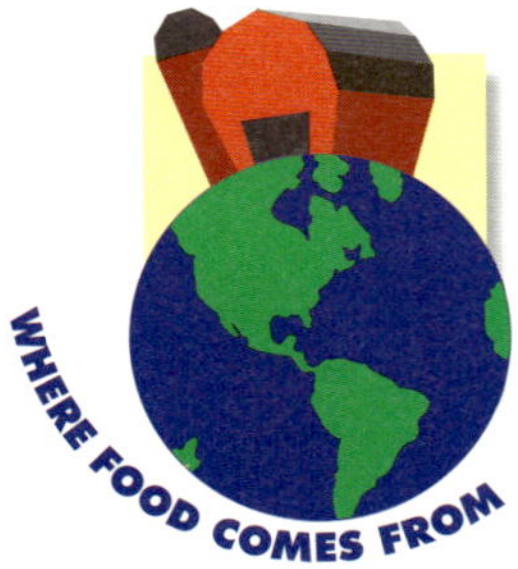

Look at the ingredient label for the many types of grains used in cereals. Look at cereal box labels and compare them. Which cereals have the most fiber? Which have the least? Which cereals contain a lot of sugar?

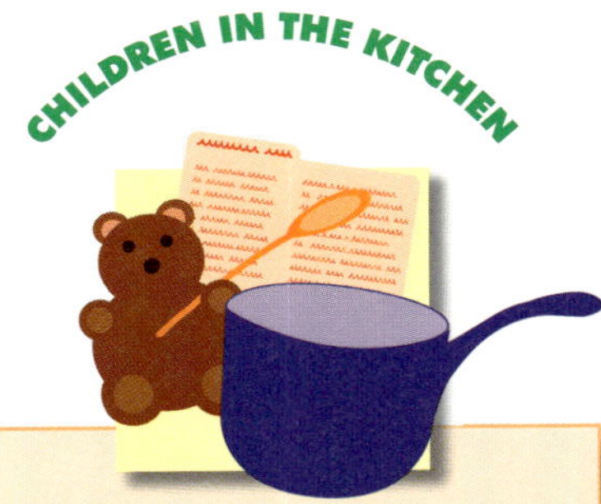

Frozen Fruit Pops

4 hours to freeze Serves: 12

It is a tasty, healthful and inexpensive way to take advantage of whatever fruit is seasonally available. Use single fruits or combine several for special "house blends."

Blender or Food Processor

- **1** ripe honeydew melon
- **2** ripe bananas
- **2** pints ripe strawberries
- ¼ cup honey or sugar

1. Help children **peel, seed,** and cut fruit into chunks. Put fruit and honey or sugar in blender in small batches and **puree**. (Pops will taste less sweet when they are frozen.)
2. **Ladle** the puree into Popsicle molds and freeze for at least 4 hours or until frozen.

Puree can be frozen in plastic ice cube trays. Poke Popsicle sticks into place when the pops are almost frozen so that the sticks will stay upright.

Nutrients per serving
one 2-oz pop

Calories	90	Saturated Fat	.1 g	Iron	.3 mg
Protein	1 g	Cholesterol	0 mg	Calcium	14 mg
Carbohydrate	23 g	Vitamin A	7 RE	Sodium	11 mg
Total Fat	.4 g	Vitamin C	55 mg	Dietary Fiber	2 g

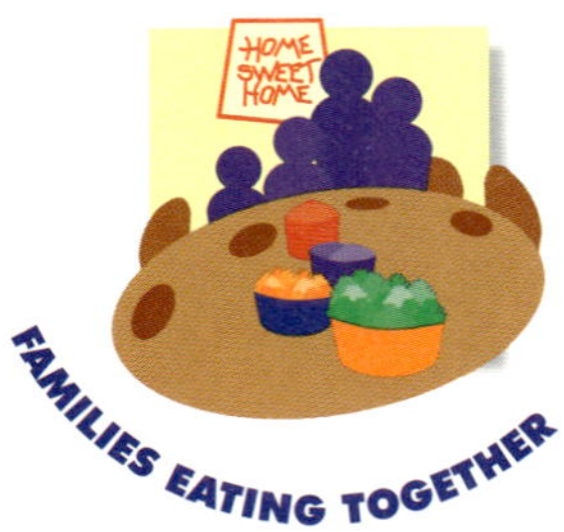

Compare the nutrition facts label of the various snacks you eat. Look at the serving size. How many cookies are in one serving? Look at the amount of fat and calories there are in one serving. Discuss which snacks make a better, more healthful choice.

School Lunch Recipe

New Macaroni and Cheese

30 minutes Serves: 10

2½ cups elbow macaroni
2½ Tbsp margarine or butter
¼ cup *plus* 2 Tbsp all-purpose flour
½ tsp ground mustard
⅛ tsp white pepper
½ tsp paprika
1 qt lowfat milk, heated
½ tsp Worcestershire sauce (optional)
2 cups lowfat cheddar cheese, shredded
2 Tbsp grated parmesan cheese (optional)
2 Tbsp fresh bread crumbs

Preheat oven to 350°F.

1. **Cook** macaroni in boiling water until firm-tender, about 8 minutes. **Drain** and **rinse** with cold water.
2. In a medium sauce pan, **melt** margarine or butter over low heat. **Add** flour, mustard, white pepper, and paprika to the melted margarine or butter and **cook** the sauce for 2 minutes, **stirring** continuously. Do not brown.
3. Slowly **add** hot milk **whisking** frequently. **Cook** over low heat, **whisking** often until it is smooth and thick.
4. **Add** Worcestershire sauce, if desired, cheddar cheese, and parmesan cheese (optional) to the white sauce. **Stir** over low heat until cheese melts.
5. **Remove** sauce from heat and **add** well-drained macaroni. **Mix** well and place in a lightly greased 13″ x 9″ x 2″ baking pan. **Cover** with foil.
6. **Bake** for 30 minutes. If desired, **sprinkle** the bread crumbs over macaroni and cheese. **Bake** uncovered for 3 to 5 minutes, until lightly browned.

Nutrients per serving
¾ cup

Calories	247	Saturated Fat	2.3 g	Iron	1.7 mg
Protein	13 g	Cholesterol	8 mg	Calcium	225 mg
Carbohydrate	34 g	Vitamin A	116 RE	Sodium	466 mg
Total Fat	6.2 g	Vitamin C	1 mg	Dietary Fiber	1 g

HOW TO EAT TO FEEL GOOD

Most American women don't have enough calcium in their diet. Depending on one's age, Americans need 2 to 3 cups of milk, or the calcium equivalent, each day. Milk, yogurt and cheese are the best sources of calcium. Lowfat and nonfat milk and lowfat and nonfat dairy products are good choices for everyone ages 2 and over.

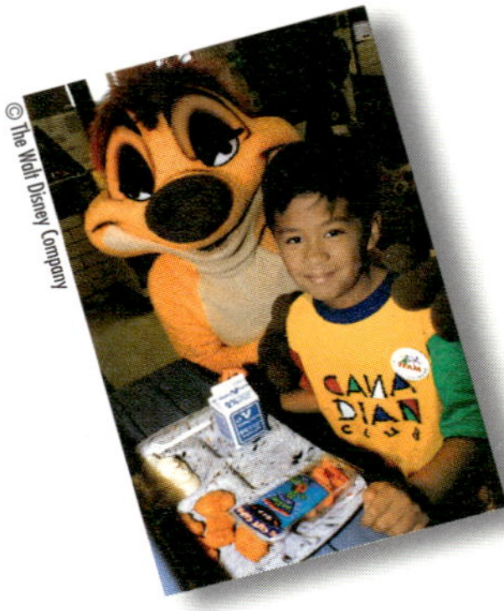
© The Walt Disney Company

THE SCHOOL LINK

Besides milk, how many types of foods at school lunch can your children count as a dairy serving? Remember to count yogurt, cheese on sandwiches, pudding and pizza cheese.

Seared Greens

15 minutes Serves: 6

You don't have to cook greens like kale or collards a long time! Lightly cooked, they retain a shiny green color, and are still chewy enough to have texture. They also keep more vitamins.

- **1½** pound of kale or collards
- **2** Tbsp olive or vegetable oil
- **4** cloves of chopped garlic
- **1** cup of water
- **¼** tsp salt
- **1** tsp black pepper
- **2** Tbsp cider vinegar

1. **Clean** the greens thoroughly and cut stems away. **Dry** well and **tear** into salad pieces or slice across the leaf into ½" pieces.
2. In a large deep pot or skillet with a cover, **saute** garlic in oil. **Add** greens in pan with 1 cup water, **cover**; **steam** for 4 minutes.
3. **Uncover, stir** constantly until greens shrink. **Add** salt and pepper and continue to stir on high until mixture is thoroughly wet. **Sprinkle** cider vinegar. **Cover; turn** off heat; **let stand** until ready to **serve**.

Nutrients per serving
1 cup

Calories	81	Saturated Fat	.4 g	Iron	2.1 mg
Protein	4 g	Cholesterol	0 mg	Calcium	159 mg
Carbohydrate	13 g	Vitamin A	1009 RE	Sodium	244 mg
Total Fat	3.1 g	Vitamin C	137 mg	Dietary Fiber	2 g

Early Vegetable and Lentil Salad

25 minutes Serves: 6

- ½ cup lentils, washed
- ½ pound new red Bliss potatoes (with skin), quartered
- ½ pound thin asparagus
- **1** cup frozen or fresh peas, shelled (in shell about 1/2 pound)
- **2** cups frozen corn
- **2** large carrots, shredded

Dressing

- **1** Tbsp fresh, chopped parsley
- **1** garlic clove, finely chopped
- **2** Tbsp red wine vinegar
- **1** Tbsp prepared mustard
- ⅓ cup olive oil

1. **Bring** 1 cup of water to a boil. **Add** the lentils and cook over low heat till tender, about 20 minutes. **Drain** the lentils.
2. **Boil** potatoes for 10-15 minutes (or microwave).
3. **Cut** the bottom 2 inches off the asparagus. Rinse the asparagus in cold water. Remove the fresh peas from their shells (optional).
4. **Steam** asparagus, peas, and corn for 3 minutes. Remove and run cold water over to stop the cooking process.
5. **For dressing: Combine** the chopped parsley, chopped garlic, vinegar and mustard in a mixing bowl. **Mix** together with a whisk, **add** the oil in a slow, steady stream.
6. **Combine** the lentils, potatoes, asparagus, peas, corn and carrots. **Toss** with dressing. Serve.

Nutrients per serving
1 cup

Calories	179	Saturated Fat	.7 g	Iron	1.9 mg
Protein	6 g	Cholesterol	0 mg	Calcium	34 mg
Carbohydrate	36 g	Vitamin A	738 RE	Sodium	73 mg
Total Fat	5.2 g	Vitamin C	19 mg	Dietary Fiber	6 g

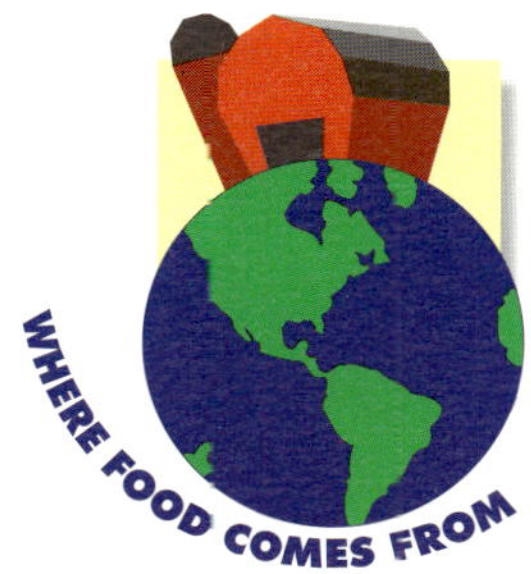

Where does milk come from? Visit a farm or dairy. Show your children milk or ice cream before it's in a package.

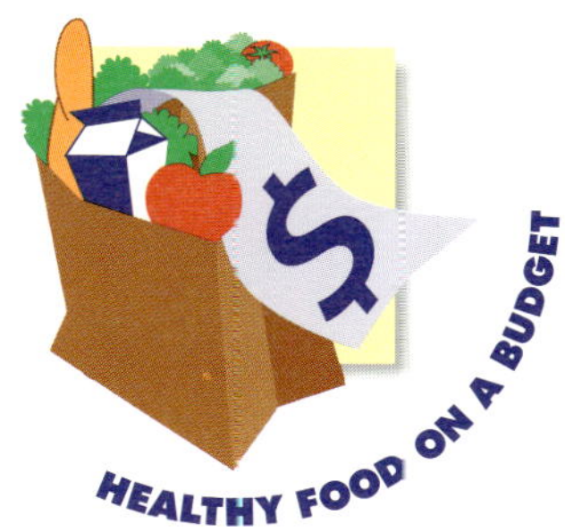

Make your own fruit yogurt dessert. Drain yogurt to make a thick cream in the refrigerator using a coffee filter in a cup. Stir in pureed fruit or jam for a nutritious and inexpensive snack.

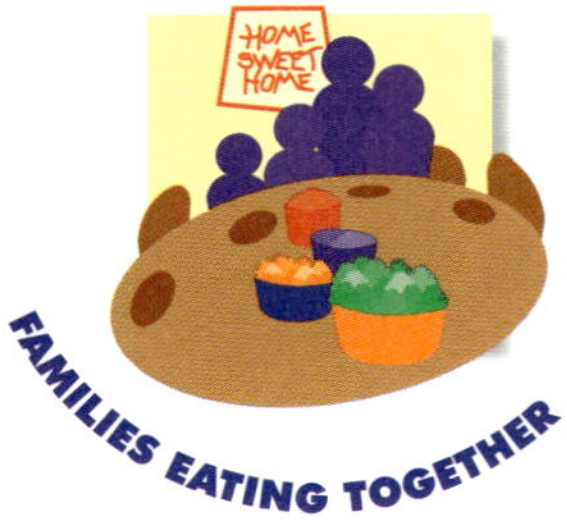

Have a dessert party at home. Serve a variety of lowfat and fat free frozen yogurts or reduced fat ice cream. Top with chopped, dried or fresh fruits, nuts and dry cereal.

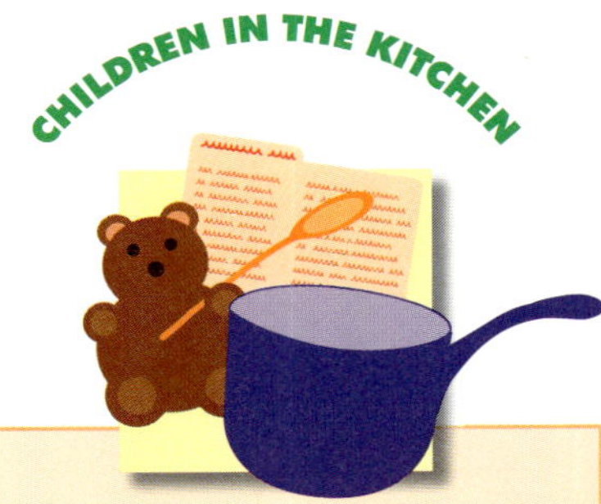

Easy Rhubarb Strawberry Crisp

25 to 30 minutes Serves: 8

If you are using fresh rhubarb, discard the leaves. If the fresh stalks are a little tough to cut, you can peel them like a carrot with a vegetable peeler.

- **2** cups fresh or frozen rhubarb, cut into 1″ pieces.
- **2** cups fresh strawberries, quartered
- **2** Tbsp lemon juice

Topping

- **1** cup topping dry oatmeal (regular or instant)
- ½ cup flour
- ½ cup brown sugar
- ½ cup white sugar
- ¼ cup margarine (½ stick)
- **1** tsp cinnamon

Extra Topping (optional)

- **1** pint vanilla lowfat **frozen** yogurt
- ¼ cup honey

1. The adult **preheats** oven to 350° F. In a large bowl, let the kids **measure** and **combine** oatmeal, flour, sugars, margarine, and cinnamon. Let them mix until the butter is soft and everything is well combined and crumbly. (Make sure everyone's hands are very clean!)
2. Have the kids **place** the fruit in a pie pan or 8″ baking dish. Sprinkle with lemon juice. **Cover** evenly with the oatmeal topping.
3. The adult **bakes** the crisp for 25 to 30 minutes, until the fruit is bubbling and the kitchen smells delicious!
4. When crisp comes out of oven, let it **cool** for 10 minutes or more, **cut** into 8 pieces. Let each child top each serving with a scoop of frozen yogurt. Drizzle honey over the top of ice cream. Enjoy!

Nutrients per serving
1 serving

Calories	245	Saturated Fat	1.2 g	Iron	1.6 mg
Protein	4 g	Cholesterol	0 mg	Calcium	57 mg
Carbohydrate	42 g	Vitamin A	73 RE	Sodium	72 mg
Total Fat	7 g	Vitamin C	4 mg	Dietary Fiber	2.7 g

Barbecued Beef

45 minutes to 1 hour Serves: 4

Serve on crusty Kaiser rolls or hamburger buns.

- **1** pound lean beef stew meat, cut into 1″ to 2″ pieces
- **1** Tbsp vegetable oil

Barbecue Sauce

- **1** cup catsup
- **1** Tbsp water
- **2** Tbsp cider vinegar
- **3** Tbsp brown sugar
- **2** tsp yellow prepared mustard
- **1** Tbsp minced onion
- **1** tsp Worcestershire Sauce (optional)
- **½** tsp chili powder
- **1** tsp cumin powder

Preheat oven to 375° F.

1. In a medium sauce pan over medium high heat, **add** oil and **brown** beef stew meat on all sides until well browned. Remove from heat and **add** remaining barbecue sauce ingredients to beef. **Stir** well.
2. **Place** into an oven proof baking dish, cover and **bake** for 45 minutes to 1 hour or until beef is tender and **shreds** easily.

Nutrients per serving
½ cup

Calories	136	Saturated Fat	1.9 g	Iron	1.4 mg
Protein	9 g	Cholesterol	26 mg	Calcium	14 mg
Carbohydrate	12 g	Vitamin A	36 RE	Sodium	394 mg
Total Fat	6.2 g	Vitamin C	5 mg	Dietary Fiber	1 g

HOW TO EAT TO FEEL GOOD

You can find healthy food choices when eating out. Remember the Food Guide Pyramid and eat the minimum number of servings from each of the Pyramid's food groups each day. Even fastfood restaurants offer healthier alternatives. Try selecting a side salad or baked potato for a change from french fries.

THE SCHOOL LINK

How are the Dietary Guidelines followed in planning school meals? Talk to your school food service staff about how food is prepared.

New Potato Salad

20 minutes Serves: 6

This salad is best served warm, but it's also fine chilled. So you can make it in advance, and refrigerate, covered, until dinner.

- **1** pound small, new (red) potatoes, quartered or halved
- **8** ounces (½ lb) small green beans, stemmed
- **2** tsp freshly-ground black pepper
- **2** green onions (scallions), trimmed and minced
- **2** Tbsp olive oil or vegetable oil
- **3** small, (ripe) tomatoes, cored
- **2** Tbsp chopped fresh parsley or basil (or 2 tsp dried)
- **¼** cup red wine vinegar
- **3** Tbsp chicken stock

1. In a large saucepan of boiling water, **cook** the potatoes until just-tender, about 15 to 20 minutes. **Cook** the green beans in a separate pan of boiling water, until just crisp-tender, about 10 to15 minutes. While they cook, **mince** the green onions (scallions) finely.
2. **Drain** potatoes and beans and place them both in a large bowl. **Add** the pepper, minced green onion, and olive oil. Gently **toss** the vegetables (they absorb more scallion and olive-oil flavors if they are still hot). Set aside to **cool**.
3. Just before serving, **add** tomato pieces, chopped herbs, vinegar, chicken stock. Again gently **toss** before serving.

Nutrients per serving
1 cup

Calories	139	Saturated Fat	.7 g	Iron	1.4 mg
Protein	3 g	Cholesterol	0 mg	Calcium	32 mg
Carbohydrate	23 g	Vitamin A	72 RE	Sodium	22 mg
Total Fat	5.0 g	Vitamin C	28 mg	Dietary Fiber	4 g

Shell Pasta Salad with Veggies

30 minutes Serves: 6

You can serve this with a purchased lowfat dressing or try this mustard vinaigrette: In a jar, combine 2 Tbsp apple cider vinegar, 2 Tbsp vegetable oil (such as olive), ¼ cup orange juice, 2 tsp mustard, 1 Tbsp grated parmesan cheese, 1 tsp garlic powder, 1 tsp dried oregano, and ¼ tsp salt. Shake to blend.

- **10** ounces of small shell pasta, cooked and chilled
- **1** sweet green pepper, diced
- **1** sweet red pepper, diced
- **1** cup of cucumber, diced
- **2** medium carrots, diced
- **1** rib of celery, diced
- **1** small red onion, diced
- **5** radishes, diced
- **¼** cup lowfat cottage cheese (optional)
- **1** 7 oz can of tuna, packed in water (optional)

1. In a large pot of water, **cook** pasta until firm-tender (*al dente*). **Drain** and **rinse** under cold water; **chill.**
2. **Dice** all vegetables and **add** to pasta. **Add** cottage cheese or tuna (optional). **Dress** with lowfat dressing. **Serve.**

Nutrients per serving
1 cup

Calories	254	Saturated Fat	0.6 g	Iron	2.4 mg
Protein	8 g	Cholesterol	1 mg	Calcium	27 mg
Carbohydrate	47 g	Vitamin A	757 RE	Sodium	26 mg
Total Fat	4 g	Vitamin C	40 mg	Dietary Fiber	4 g

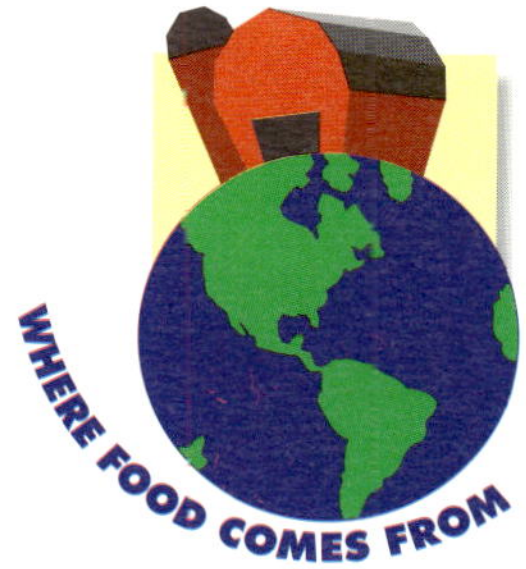

At a local restaurant, ask to talk with the chef. Ask the chef what foods are lower in fat and if the restaurant highlights healthful menu choices.

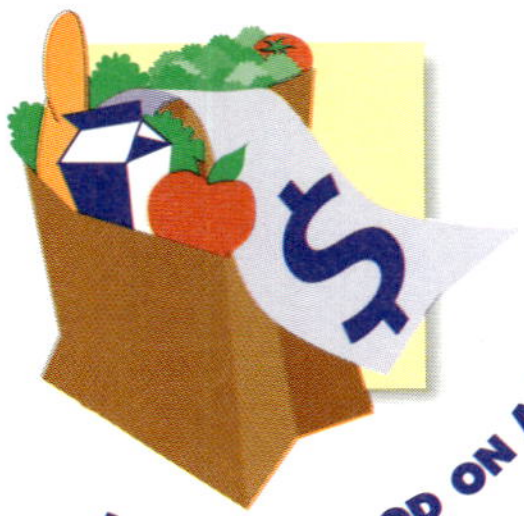

HEALTHY FOOD ON A BUDGET

Planning ahead can save money. To bypass fastfood restaurants, make quick snacks and ready-to-go foods. Wrapping up some cheese and crackers with a piece of fruit, or bean burritos and a can of juice can save you time and money when you are out of the house.

CHILDREN IN THE KITCHEN

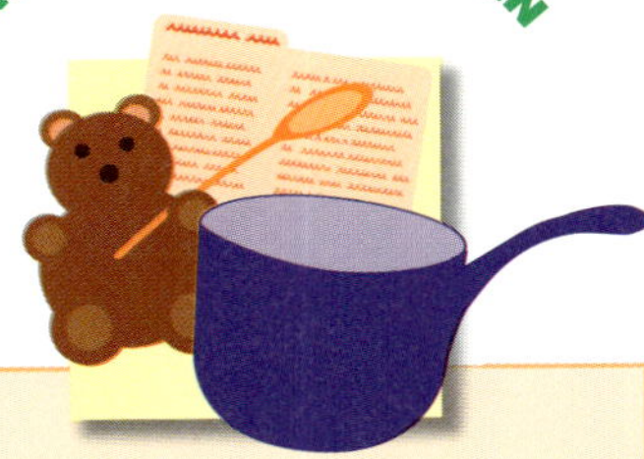

Cinco de Mayo Nachos

20 minutes Serves: 4

"Cinco de Mayo" means the 5th of May. It is the anniversary date for the independence of Mexico, and it is celebrated throughout that country, by Mexican-Americans here, and by anyone who loves Mexican culture. If you make this treat with children, have one child look up the history of "Cinco de Mayo" to share with everyone. These days, you can buy excellent salsas in the supermarket. Look for those that are low in sodium. If you want to make fresh salsa, though, it's easy; see the recipe in July (pg 72).

- **1** cup onions, finely diced
- **2** cloves fresh garlic, minced
- **1** Tbsp fresh or canned jalapeno peppers, chopped
- **1** whole green bell pepper, diced
- **1** lb can cooked red kidney beans, black beans, or pinto beans, drained and rinsed
- **1** 10 ounce bag baked (lowfat) corn (tortilla) chips
- **1** fresh tomato, diced
- **3** ounces shredded lowfat mozzarella

Toppings: more onions, nonfat sour cream, salsa, chopped olives (all optional)

Preheat oven to 350° F.

If kids are old enough to hold a knife, they can **dice** the onions (don't cry!) and garlic, and **chop** the jalapenos.

(continued on back of card)

Cinco de Mayo Nachos, continued

1. An adult **heats** a non-stick pan (or use 1 tsp oil in regular pan) to **saute** onions on medium high until clear. **Add** garlic and **saute** for one minute. **Add** beans, pepper, and jalapenos to pan, **cook** and stir for about 10 minutes.
2. The adult **takes** the pan off the stove, **transfers** the contents to a bowl. The kids **mash** bean mixture until smooth, only adding water if necessary to make puree smooth.
3. The kids **place** chips on a baking sheet. With adult supervision, kids can **spread** beans, onions and pepper mixture evenly on top of tortilla chips. Kids can then **sprinkle** cheese and diced tomatoes. **Bake** until cheese melts, about 10 minutes.
4. Kids can help **put** vegetables, more chopped onions, and toppings around serving dish. Each guest, child or adult, **tops** his or her own nacho.

Nutrients per serving

Calories	412	Saturated Fat	2 g	Iron	1.3 mg
Protein	18 g	Cholesterol	7 mg	Calcium	286 mg
Carbohydrate	78 g	Vitamin A	56 RE	Sodium	721 mg
Total Fat	5 g	Vitamin C	26 mg	Dietary Fiber	11 g

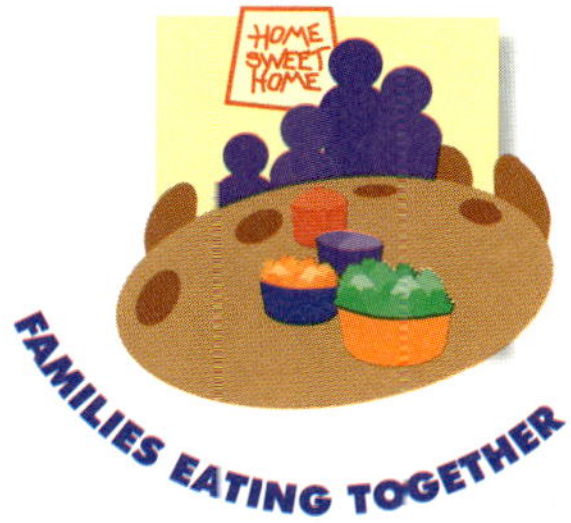

When you eat out, try new tastes. Are there seafood or ethnic restaurants that might offer new foods and foods with different flavors that you don't usually prepare at home?

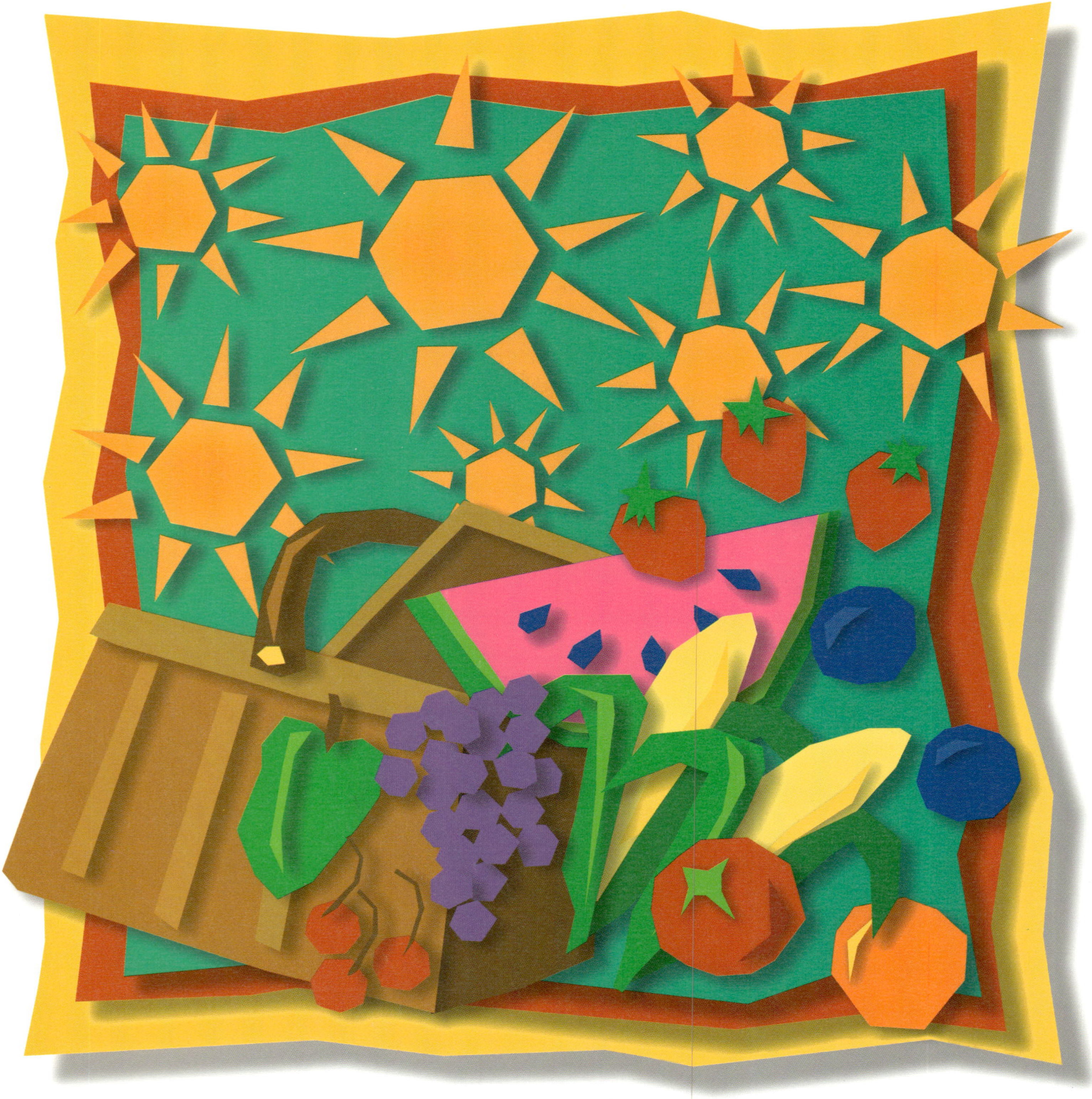

Summer

In the summer, nearly everything comes into full bloom: flowers, fruits, kids. It's the season of play. And seasonal fruits and vegetables, inexpensive and at the peak of flavor, make it easy to eat as well.

Fruits are ripe and luscious. Strawberries, blueberries, and other berries make their brief appearance at their freshest, cherries are red and sweet, grapes are in, and every kind of melon is sweet and juicy: cantaloupe, honeydew, watermelon. In some markets, fresh apricots are available; sometimes, figs, peaches and plums are ripe. For citrus fruits, Valencia oranges are at their peak.

Summer vegetables are a joy to behold. Cucumbers, eggplant, green snap beans,

Summer Chef Teams Included:

Monique Barbear, Tom Douglas, Paul O'Connell, Nick Zakharoff, Lucie Costa, Ronald De Santis, and Damian Martineau

fresh lima beans, and lettuces of all varieties are in season. If you like okra, now is the time to find it fresh. Peppers in all colors, green and yellow and red, are available. Summer squash is in. So are red ripe tomatoes, and, that most summery of treats, corn on the cob. Summer vegetables reach their peak of flavor and nutrition, and become more affordable, at the same time.

This is a fun time to enjoy summer weather and eat foods outside. We include a summer grilled chicken salad and a garden vegetable rice salad recipe (see pg 66 and pg 71) for your picnics.

As always, the foundation of the Food Guide Pyramid, the Breads, Cereal, Rice, and Pasta Group, is available. So are the Milk, Yogurt, and Cheese Group, and the Meat Poultry, Fish, Dry Beans, Eggs, and Nuts Group. If you fish in the summer, you'll bring home a good source of lowfat protein.

Our recipes take advantage of summertime bargains. When tomatoes are fresh and inexpensive, try Spaghetti with Marinated Tomatoes (pg 65) and Homemade Salsa (pg 72). When fruit is ripe, our Quick Summer Fruit Shortcake (pg 68) and Fruit Yogurt Shake (pg 73) make good use of them. So does Watermelon Ice (pg 77). And many others.

In Season:

Vegetables:
Cabbage, carrots, celery, cucumbers, eggplant, green beans, lima beans, lettuce, okra, onions, peppers, potatoes, squash, sweet corn, tomatoes.

Fruits:
Apricots, berries, cantaloupes, cherries, figs, grapes, honeydew melons, lemons, nectarines, peaches, plums, strawberries, Valencia oranges, watermelons.

Also:
All dairy, meats and poultry products, most fish and shellfish.

HOW TO EAT TO FEEL GOOD

Spaghetti with Marinated Tomatoes

15 minutes Serves: 8

- **1** lb. cooked spaghetti
- **1½** lb. fresh tomatoes (or whole canned tomatoes)
- **3** garlic cloves
- A dozen fresh basil leaves (or ¼ cup chopped fresh parsley)
- **½** cup olive oil

1. **Blanch** fresh tomatoes in boiling water for a few seconds and **remove** peel; **cut** tomatoes in half and **remove** seeds; **slice** tomatoes into thin strips.
2. **Place** tomatoes in a bowl and **add** crushed garlic, chopped basil and olive oil.
3. Cook spaghetti according to directions on the box. **Toss** with marinated tomatoes. If desired, **top** with grated Parmesan cheese. **Serve.**

Nutrients per serving
1 cup

Calories	159	Saturated Fat	1 g	Iron	1.2 mg
Protein	3.5	Cholesterol	0 mg	Calcium	11 mg
Carbohydrate	20 g	Vitamin A	55 RE	Sodium	64 mg
Total Fat	7.4 g	Vitamin C	17 mg	Dietary Fiber	2 g

Balance the food you eat with physical activity: maintain or improve your weight. Approximately one-third of American children and adults are overweight. Being more physically active helps your body get the most benefit from a good diet. Any type of exercise uses calories and can be helpful in a weight loss program. Being active helps.

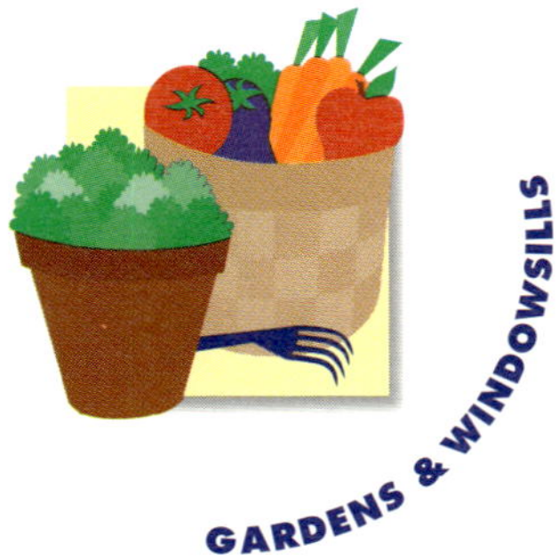

Have you tried growing your own herbs? They're simple to grow. Buy the herb seeds or seedlings (small plants) from a nursery or the gardening department of a store. Herbs grow best in average garden soil with plenty of sun and occasional watering. They grow well on a sunny windowsill in containers, as well as outdoors. Herbs are easy to harvest—just pick the leaves. To dry herbs, hang branches upside down in a cool, dark place. Pull off the dried leaves and store in jars with lids. Great to use for flavoring in place of added fat or salt.

Summer Grilled Chicken Salad

30 minutes Serves: 4

French bread is nice with this dish.

- **4** Chicken thighs, skinless
- **1½** tsp seasoned salt for grilling (optional)
- **2** ears corn-on-the-cob, fresh with husk (frozen or canned may be used)
- **1** 10-oz package frozen lima beans, cooked
- **1** small red bell pepper, diced
- **1** 16 oz can black beans, rinsed
- **1** Tbsp cilantro, chopped
- **¼** cup Italian lowfat salad dressing

1. **Start** grill. **Sprinkle** the seasoned salt (optional) over the chicken thighs and **grill** them until done over medium high heat, about 10–15 minutes or until juices run clear.
2. **Remove** the chicken from the grill and allow to **cool**, then **remove** the meat from the bone and **dice** into large pieces.
3. While the chicken is cooling, **place** the fresh corn-on-the-cob still in the husk on the **grill** for 15-20 minutes.

   Remove the corn kernels from the cob.
4. **Combine** diced chicken, corn kernels. and remaining ingredients. **Toss** with dressing and coat well.

Nutrients per serving
1 cup

Calories	285	Saturated Fat	1.3 g	Iron	2.8 mg
Protein	17g	Cholesterol	33 mg	Calcium	45 mg
Carbohydrate	25 g	Vitamin A	94 RE	Sodium	329 mg
Total Fat	5.5 g	Vitamin C	30 mg	Dietary Fiber	6 g

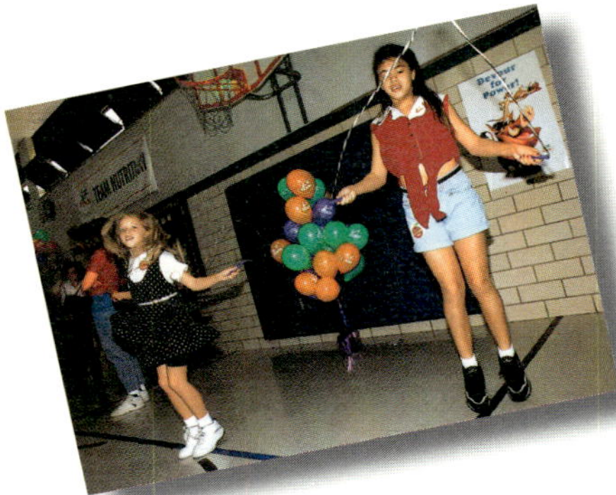

Peach Cobbler

35 minutes **Serves: 4**

You can substitute any fruit in season: blueberries or strawberries work well.

- **4** very ripe peaches, peeled and sliced (or frozen, or canned peaches)
- **2** tablespoons sugar
- **1⅓** cups all-purpose flour
- ¼ cup sugar
- **2** tsp baking powder
- **1½** Tbsp margarine or butter
- ½ cup lowfat milk

1. **Toss** the 2 Tbsp sugar with the peaches; place in a 1½ quart ovenproof dish.
2. To make the dough, **place** the flour, sugar and baking powder in a bowl; **add** the margarine and milk; stir until well mixed.
3. **Place** the dish with peaches into the oven. **Heat** until warm and the sugar starts to melt.
4. **Drop** the dough on top by spoonfuls. **Bake** in oven for about 35 minutes or until the fruit begins to bubble and the topping is slightly brown. Let it cool a bit, and **serve**.

Nutrients per serving
1/2 cup

Calories	312	Saturated Fat	1.1 g	Iron	2.3 mg
Protein	6 g	Cholesterol	1 mg	Calcium	184 mg
Carbohydrate	62 g	Vitamin A	122 RE	Sodium	260 mg
Total Fat	5 g	Vitamin C	6 mg	Dietary Fiber	3 g

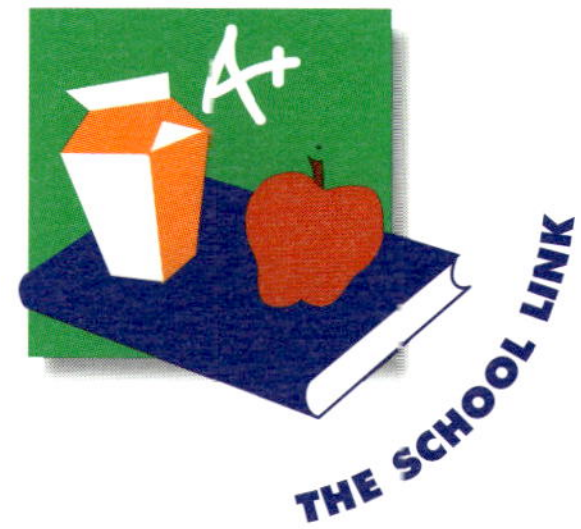

Getting exercise at school is important. Encourage your children to participate in active play at recess. Ask your school principal to offer regular physical education classes.

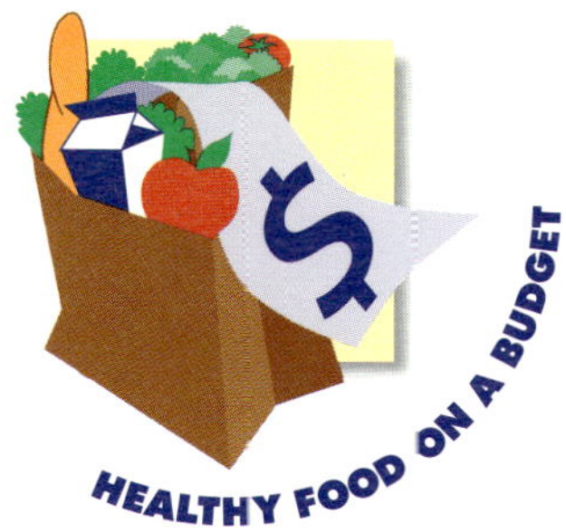

Drink plenty of water and other fluids. Water, juices and milk are better nutrition choices than soft drinks.

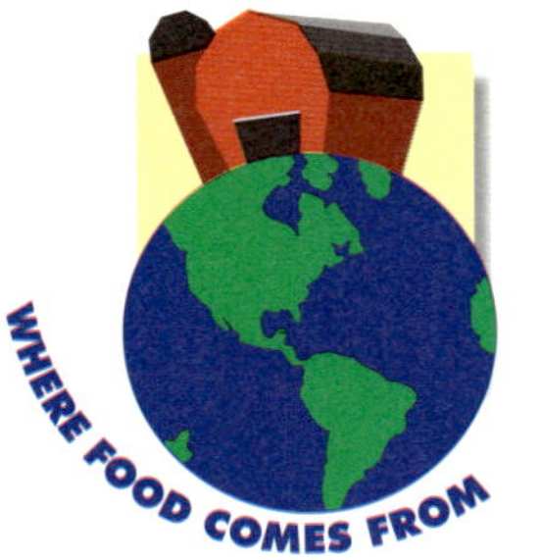

Get exercise while choosing spring fruits. Either go berry picking at a farm or take a walk through an outdoor market.

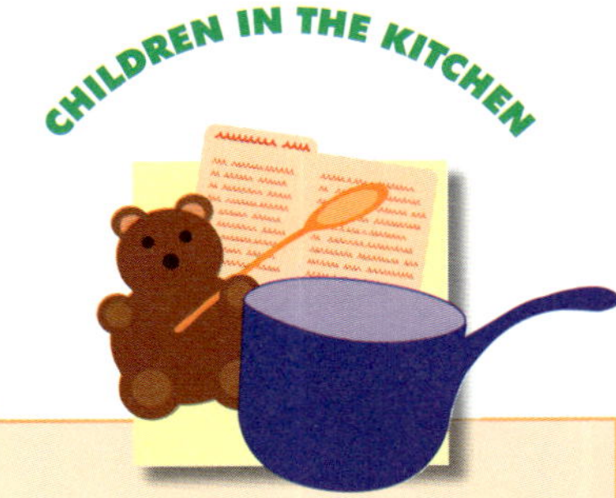

Quick Summer Fruit Shortcake

20 minutes Serves: 4

Frozen or canned fruit can be used in this recipe, too!

- **1** pint strawberries, cleaned and hulled
- **1** cup grapes, seedless, cleaned and halved
- **2** each peaches, diced
- **3** Tbsp sugar
- **¼** cup orange juice
- **4** slices angel food cake

1. The kids can help with this step. If using strawberries, **quarter** them first. **Combine** berries, grapes, peaches, sugar and orange juice in a large bowl. **Mix** well. **Cover** with plastic wrap; **refrigerate** for 20 minutes.
2. Kids **put** one slice of cake on each plate; then portion the fruit and juices from the bowl on top of each slice of cake. **Serve.**

Nutrients per serving
1 serving

Calories	148	Saturated Fat	.1 g	Iron	.3 mg
Protein	2 g	Cholesterol	0 mg	Calcium	46 mg
Carbohydrate	36 g	Vitamin A	27 RE	Sodium	210 mg
Total Fat	.4 g	Vitamin C	9 mg	Dietary Fiber	2g

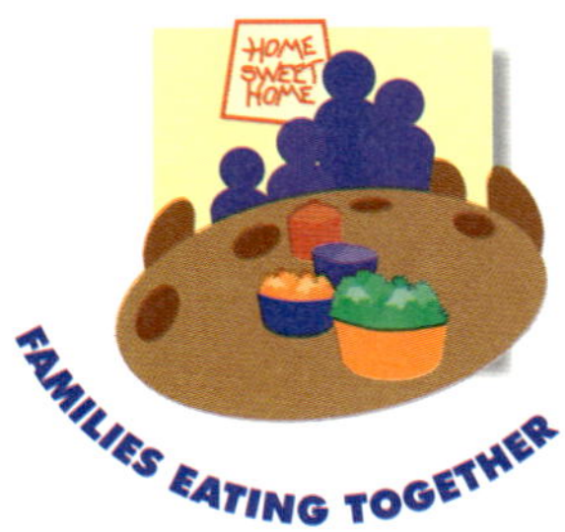

On the weekend take a family hike with a snack in a backpack or bag. Remember variety. Dry cereals, dried fruits, nuts and apple slices won't weight the pack down. Encourage exercise — take a family walk after dinner.

School Lunch Recipe

Chicken Stir-Fry

25 minutes Serves: 8

Variation: Use cubes of beef, pork or turkey for another stir-fry! Or just add vegetables and tofu (bean curd), for a vegetable stir-fry!

- **2** Tbsp cornstarch
- ¼ cup low-sodium soy sauce
- ⅛ tsp ground ginger
- **2** tsp granulated garlic
- ½ tsp white pepper
- **1** Tbsp sesame oil (optional)
- 1¾ cups chicken broth
- ½ cup water
- **1** Tbsp vegetable oil
- **1** lb skinless, boneless chicken breasts, diced
- **1** Tbsp vegetable oil

Mixed vegetables:

- 1½ cups fresh carrots, peeled, diced
- ⅓ cup onions, diced
- 2½ cups fresh broccoli florets, or **2** cups frozen mixed oriental vegetables

Sauce:

1. **Dissolve** cornstarch in soy sauce. **Add** ginger, garlic, pepper, and sesame oil (optional) to cornstarch mixture and **whisk** to blend.
2. In saucepan, **bring** chicken broth and water to a boil.
3. Slowly **add** cornstarch mixture, **whisking** continuously until combined. **Return** sauce to a boil. **Reduce** heat to simmer and **continue** cooking until sauce is smooth and thick, about 3 to 5 minutes. **Remove** from heat.

continued on next card

HOW TO EAT TO FEEL GOOD

Fill the gap between knowing and doing. Most of us know that variety is important. Make it a goal for your family to try at least one new fruit each month. Make fruit easy for your kids to see and reach. Try a fruit bowl on the table.

THE SCHOOL LINK

Ask your children how many fruits they had today. Do they need to eat more fruit according to the Food Guide Pyramid? Remember, fruit is an easy snack. It works well for picnics and school snacks. Bananas, raisins and apples pack well.

Chicken Stir-Fry, continued

Chicken:

4. In a medium skillet, **heat** 1Tbsp oil over medium-high heat. **Add** chicken and **saute** over medium heat for 5 to 10 minutes until no signs of pink remain. **Remove** chicken from heat, **cover** and **set aside.**

Vegetables:

5. In the same skillet, **heat** 1 Tbsp of oil over medium-high heat. If using fresh vegetables, **saute** carrots over medium heat for 4 minutes. **Add** onions and cook for 1 minute. **Add** broccoli and **cook** for 2 more minutes. If **using** frozen vegetables, **add** vegetables to oil and **cook** over medium heat until tender, about 3 minutes.

Combine:

6. **Add** cooked chicken and reserved sauce to vegetables and **toss** to thoroughly **coat.** It's time to eat!

Nutrients per serving
¾ cup

Calories	149	Saturated Fat	1.1 g	Iron	1.0 mg
Protein	16 g	Cholesterol	33 mg	Calcium	30 mg
Carbohydrate	7 g	Vitamin A	665 RE	Sodium	323 mg
Total Fat	6.3 g	Vitamin C	22 mg	Dietary Fiber	2 g

Garden Vegetable Rice Salad

40 minutes Serves: 12

- **2** cups long grain rice
- **4½** cups water
- **1** bay leaf
- **2** lemons
- **2** tsp margarine
- **2** Tbsp olive oil

- ½ cup fresh basil, shredded
- ½ cup zucchini, diced
- ½ cup yellow squash, diced
- ¼ cup red pepper, diced
- ½ cup eggplant, diced
- ½ cup tomato, diced
- **2** Tbsp olive oil
- **1** clove garlic
- ¼ cup fresh basil
- Juice of **1** lemon

1. **Bring water to a boil** in saucepan. **Add** the bay leaf, one lemon cut in half, rice, and margarine. **Turn down heat** to low and **cover. Cook** for approximately 20 minutes until the rice is tender. **Place** cooked rice in refrigerator to cool. **Discard** bay leaf and lemon halves.
2. **Heat** a large skillet over medium heat. **Place** 2 Tbsp olive oil in the skillet and add the zucchini and yellow squash. **Stir-fry** for 8 minutes over medium heat **stirring** occasionally. Add half of basil and remove to serving bowl.
3. Return to skillet and **add** the red pepper, eggplant, tomato, and garlic along with the remaining olive oil. **Cook** for 5-10 minutes over medium heat until the eggplant is tender, but not mushy.
4. Toss all vegetables together with remaining basil and juice of one lemon. **Add** rice to vegetables and toss together for a great summer salad.

Nutrients per serving
1 cup

Calories	176	Saturated Fat	.8 g	Iron	1.5 mg
Protein	3 g	Cholesterol	0 mg	Calcium	37 mg
Carbohydrate	30 g	Vitamin A	41 RE	Sodium	12 mg
Total Fat	5.6 g	Vitamin C	23 mg	Dietary Fiber	2 g

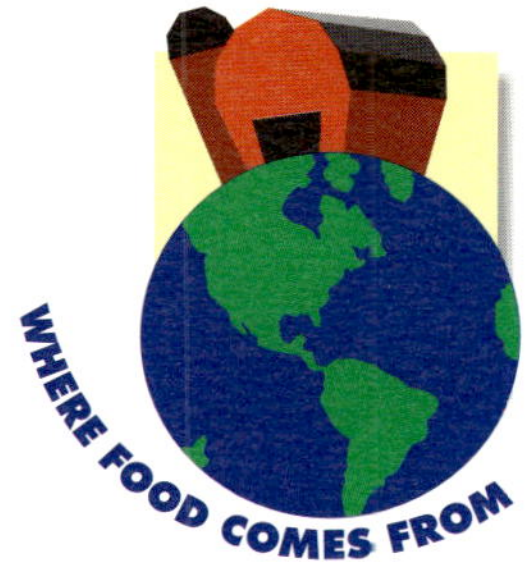

Show children where orange juice comes from —give each child a plastic juicer and an orange. Have the children roll the oranges, then you cut in half... let them make their own cup of juice for their snack.

HEALTHY FOOD ON A BUDGET

Banana pops! Give each child half a banana and a Popsicle stick. Let the children peel it, insert the stick in the banana, then roll the banana in granola cereal. Place the "banana pop" in a cup or holder, and place in the freezer for several hours before serving!

Homemade Salsa

15 minutes Serves: 6

- **1** cup fresh tomatoes, diced
- **½** cup corn kernels, fresh or frozen
- **½** cup onion, diced
- **1** Tbsp (or less) jalapeno peppers, chopped
- **2** Tbsp lime juice
- **2** cloves fresh garlic, finely diced

1. **Combine** all of the above ingredients
2. **Serve** with lowfat baked tortilla (corn) chips, or fresh veggies, cut up.

Nutrients per serving
½ cup

Calories	33	Saturated Fat	0 g	Iron	.4 mg
Protein	1 g	Cholesterol	0 mg	Calcium	8 mg
Carbohydrate	8 g	Vitamin A	42 RE	Sodium	26 mg
Total Fat	.4 g	Vitamin C	15 mg	Dietary Fiber	1 g

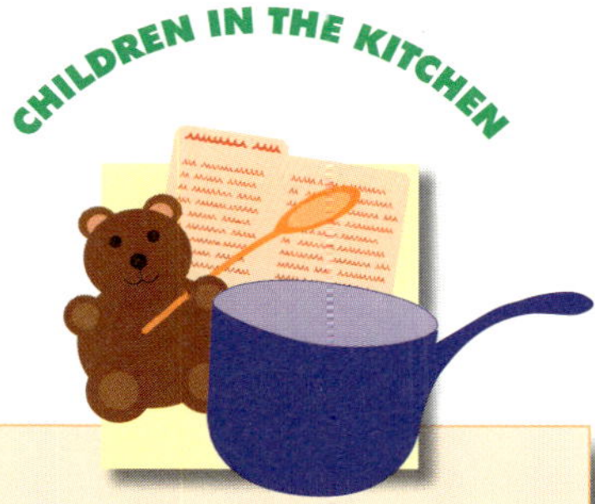

Fruit Yogurt Shake

About 10 minutes Serves: 2

1 cup fruit (peaches, strawberries, bananas), cut up
4 scoops (1 1/3 cups) nonfat frozen yogurt
2 cups skim milk, ice cold
2 Tbsp sugar

1. Have kids cut up fruit—carefully. Have them put all ingredients into blender, close top, then **puree**.
2. Kids **pour** into chilled glasses. **Serve** with straws. Cool!

Nutrients per serving
1 cup

Calories	291	Saturated Fat	0.3 g	Iron	.3 mg
Protein	12 g	Cholesterol	16 mg	Calcium	427 mg
Carbohydrate	53 g	Vitamin A	208 RE	Sodium	201 mg
Total Fat	0.6 g	Vitamin C	7 mg	Dietary Fiber	1 g

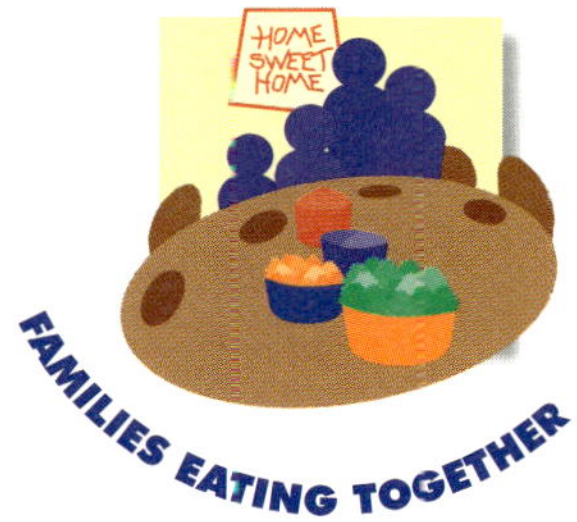

Have a family fruit festival. Layer fruit with lowfat yogurt in dishes. Serve a fruit salad. Try a frui-shake.

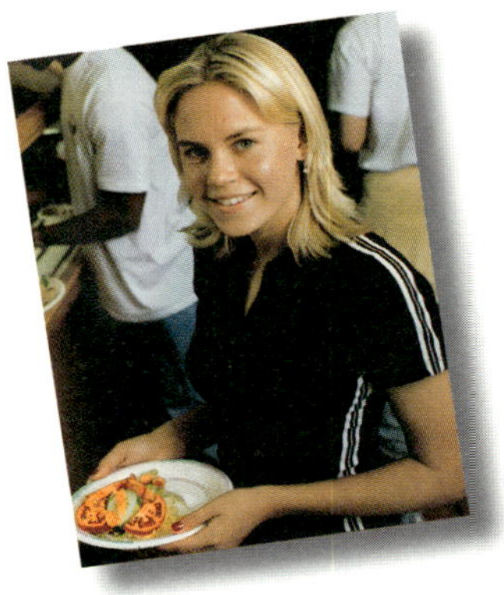

HOW TO EAT TO FEEL GOOD

Be a "choosy chewer." Consider how preparing food makes a difference in nutrition. Choose to use less sugar, fat and salt in your recipes. Use herbs and spices for seasoning.

Garden Fresh Tomato Sauce

15 minutes Serves: 4

This makes a delicious simple sauce for pasta.

- **3** cups chopped tomatoes
- **1** Tbsp garlic powder
- **1** Tbsp onion powder
- **2** fresh basil leaves, chopped (or ¼ tsp dried basil)
- **2** stems fresh oregano chopped (or ¼ tsp dried oregano)
- **2** stems fresh parsley, chopped (or ¼ tsp dried parsley)
- ½ tsp fennel seed
- ⅛ tsp black pepper

1. In a saucepan **combine** all sauce ingredients.
2. **Simmer** on medium heat for 15 minutes or until tomatoes are soft. Serve over cooked pasta.

Variations using Sauce:

To make a hearty minestrone:
Add 2 cups of chicken broth, 1 cup of cooked macaroni, 1 cup of any vegetable or left-over vegetables such as cooked and diced carrots, green beans, celery and turn your sauce into a meal. Serve with a slice of crusty bread and cheese.

To make Chili:
Add ½ pound of cooked lean ground meat, 1 cup of pinto beans, 1 tsp of chili powder, ¼ tsp cumin and one dash of Tabasco sauce. Serve in a soup bowl, sprinkle with cheddar cheese and add corn chips.

Nutrients per serving
1 cup

Calories	47	Saturated Fat	.1 g	Iron	.9 mg
Protein	2 g	Cholesterol	0 mg	Calcium	25 mg
Carbohydrate	11 g	Vitamin A	88 RE	Sodium	305 mg
Total Fat	.6 g	Vitamin C	27 mg	Dietary Fiber	2 g

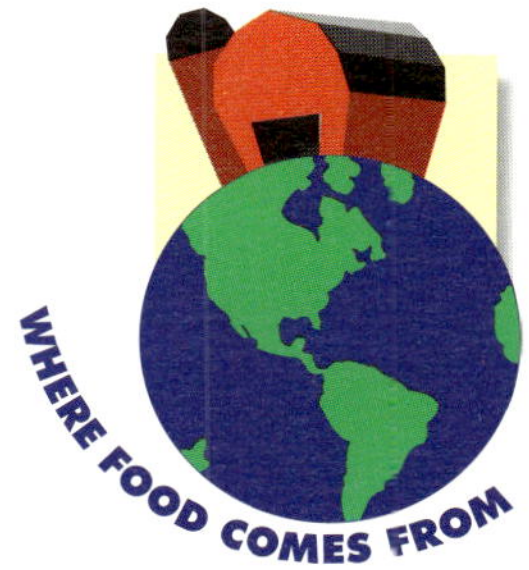

Snappy Green Beans with Basil Dip

20 minutes Serves: 4

- ½ pound (8 oz) fresh green beans, washed and stemmed
- ⅓ cup lowfat mayonnaise
- **2** Tbsp 1% milk
- **1** tsp onion powder
- **1** Tbsp fresh basil, chopped

Seasonings to taste

1. **Mix** all ingredients except green beans.
2. **Put** in small bowl placed in center of serving platter: surround by green beans. **Serve.**

Nutrients per serving, dip only
2 Tbsp

Calories	66	Saturated Fat	1.3 g	Iron	0 mg
Protein	0 g	Cholesterol	0 mg	Calcium	12 mg
Carbohydrate	2 g	Vitamin A	7 RE	Sodium	138 mg
Total Fat	6.2 g	Vitamin C	0 mg	Dietary Fiber	0 g

Make a chart on where food comes from. Using corn as an example: Show the seed, how it is grown, how it is harvested, how it is brought to a production plant or delivered to storage or a food distribution center, bought at a market, and then prepared in different ways at home! Use props like seeds, drawings or real cornstalks, and fresh, canned, or frozen corn and discuss the various ways corn can be served.

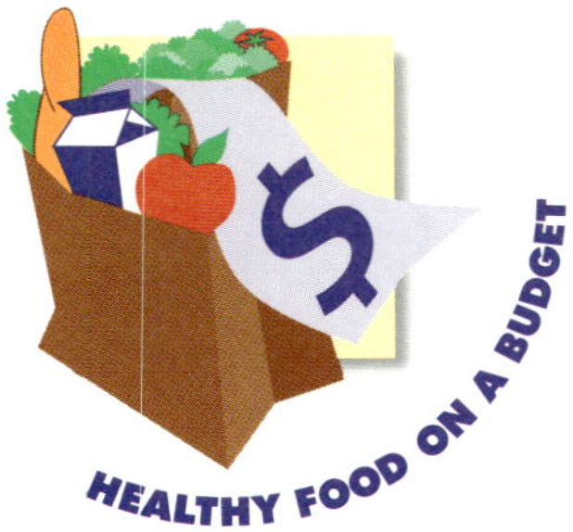

Planning ahead saves time, effort and money, and it helps increase variety and balance in the diet. Plan meals for the week. Make a shopping list before you go to the store. Consider store "specials" and use food coupons in planning your list.

Grilled Corn-on-the-Cob with Pepper Seasoning

10 to15 minutes Serves: 4

To roast bell pepper, place on baking sheet; broil in oven until blistered and charred. Put in heavy plastic or paper bag, seal; let set for 20 minutes. Peel skin; don't worry if all the charred parts don't come off. (If you don't have time to roast the pepper, purchase roasted peppers, or omit peppers entirely.)

- **1** red bell pepper, roasted, peeled, seeded and diced (optional)
- **1** Tbsp margarine
- **¼** cup chopped fresh cilantro (optional)
- **2** Tbsp chopped green onions (scallions) or chives, snipped
- **¼** tsp salt
- **⅛** tsp freshly ground black pepper
- **⅛** tsp Tabasco (optional)
- **4** ears fresh sweet corn

Preheat the outdoor grill.

1. In a blender or food processor, **combine** the red pepper, margarine, green onions and cilantro (optional). **Add** salt, pepper and Tabasco, if desired.
2. **Husk** and clean the corn. **Place** each ear individually in the center of a piece of aluminum foil, shiny side up. **Coat** each ear with a quarter of the pepper seasoning mixture. **Wrap** the foil around the corn, making sure the ear is well sealed by the foil. (**Refrigerate** until ready to grill).
3. **Place** corn on grill near the edges or cooler areas. **Grill** until tender, turning frequently, about 10 to 15 minutes. Carefully **unwrap** the corn and **serve**.

Nutrients per serving
1 serving of corn

Calories	103	Saturated Fat	.6 g	Iron	.5 mg
Protein	3 g	Cholesterol	0 mg	Calcium	4 mg
Carbohydrate	17 g	Vitamin A	61 RE	Sodium	192 mg
Total Fat	3.9 g	Vitamin C	6 mg	Dietary Fiber	3 g

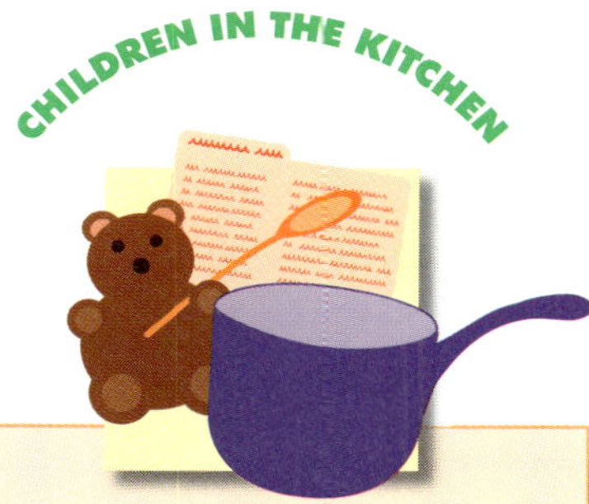

Watermelon Ice

5 minutes Serves: 1

1 cup watermelon, cubed
½ cup cracked ice
3 Tbsp of sugar

Squeezed juice of 1 lime

1. In a blender, have kids **place** ice cubes, sugar, lime and watermelon. **Process** until well blended.
2. **Place** into freezer until slushy and ready to serve. **Enjoy!**

Nutrients per serving
6 oz

Calories	102	Saturated Fat	0 g	Iron	.2 mg
Protein	1 g	Cholesterol	0 mg	Calcium	9 mg
Carbohydrate	26 g	Vitamin A	28 RE	Sodium	3 mg
Total Fat	.3 g	Vitamin C	13 mg	Dietary Fiber	0 g

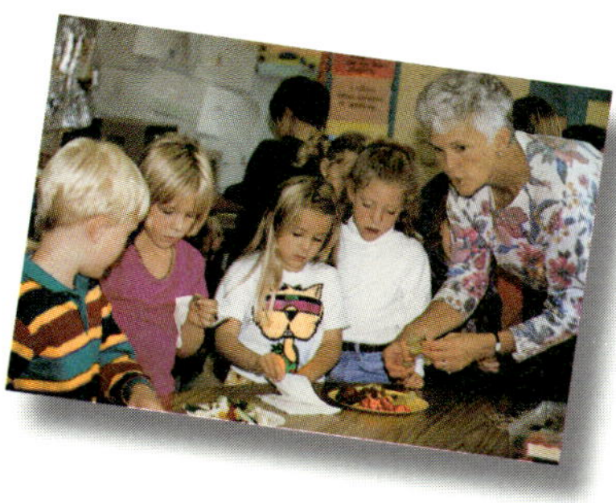

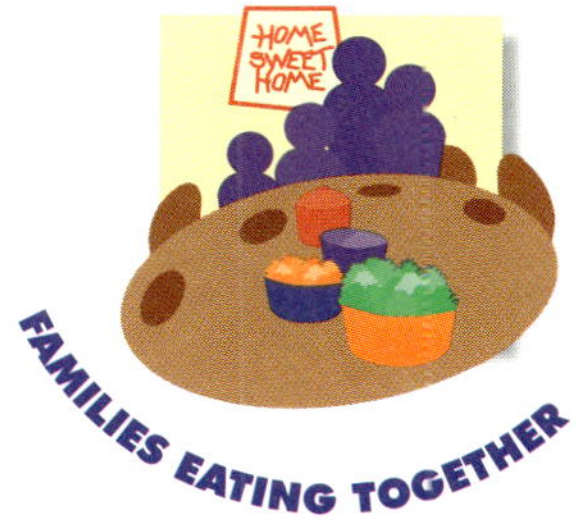

Eat outside for a change. Have each family member choose and prepare a healthy picnic meal, and help cook it.

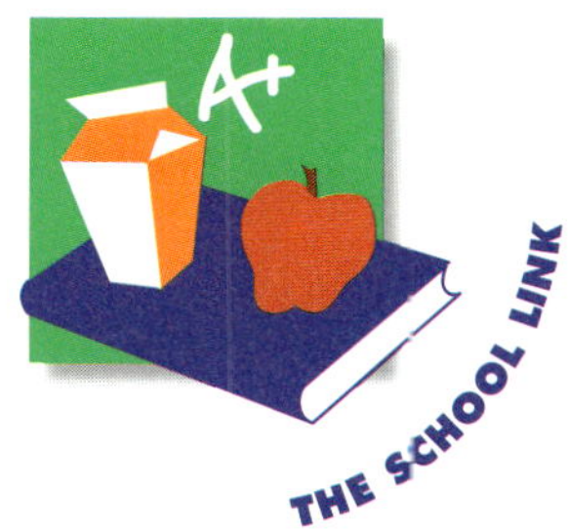

Plan a menu for your school field trip: a brownbag lunch that reflects the Food Guide Pyramid. Can you put in an extra grain or vegetable?

Resources

Contents

Understanding the USDA'S Food Guide Pyramid

No one food gives you all the nutrients you need to stay healthy, so it is best to eat a variety of different foods every day.

Use the Food Guide Pyramid to help you eat better every day.... The Dietary Guidelines' way.

Start with plenty of Breads, Cereals, Rice, and Pasta, Vegetables, and Fruits. Add 2 to 3 servings from the Milk group and 2 to 3 servings from the Meat group.

Go easy on fats, oils, and sweets, the foods in the small tip of the Pyramid.

Nutrients are found in all foods.

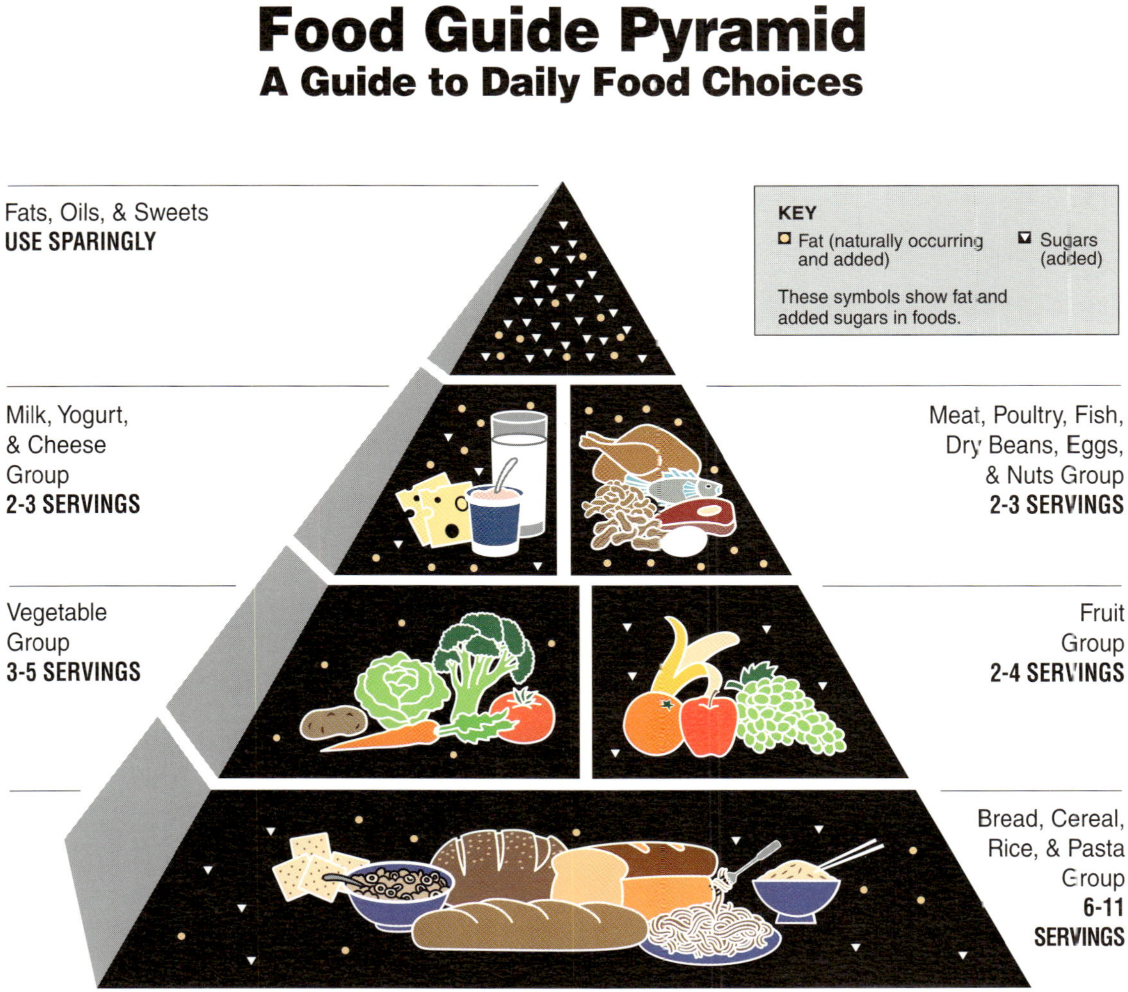

Source: U.S. Department of Agriculture/U.S. Department of Health and Human Services

What Counts as 1 Serving?

Bread, Cereals, Rice, and Pasta
1 slice of bread
1/2 cup of cooked cereal, rice or pasta
1 ounce of ready-to-eat cereal

Vegetables
1 cup of raw, leafy vegetables
1/2 cup of other vegetable, cooked or chopped raw
3/4 cup of vegetable juice

Fruits
1 medium whole fruit
1/2 cup of chopped, cooked, or canned fruit
3/4 cup of juice

Milk
1 cup of milk
8 ounces of yogurt
1-1/2 ounces of natural cheese
2 ounces of processed cheese

Meat, Poultry, Fish, Dry Beans, Eggs and Nuts
2-3 ounces of cooked meat, poultry, or fish (3 ounces of meat is about the same size as a deck of cards)

1/2 cup of cooked dry beans or 1 egg, 2 tablespoons of peanut butter or 1/3 cup of nuts count as 1 ounce of meat (about 1/3 serving)

Fats, Oils, and Sweets
Use sparingly. These are foods such as salad dressings, cream, butter, margarine, sugars, soft drinks, and candies. Go easy on these foods because they have a lot of calories from fat and sugars, but few nutrients.

SAMPLE DIETS FOR A DAY AT 3 CALORIE LEVELS

	Women & some older adults	Children, teen girls, active women, most men	Teen boys & active men
Calorie Levels*	**Lower** about **1,600**	**Moderate** about **2,200**	**Higher** about **2,800**
Bread group	6	9	11
Vegetable group	3	4	5
Fruit group	2	3	4
Milk group	2–3**	2–3**	2–3**
Meat group (total ounces)	2 (5 ounces)	2 (6 ounces)	3 (7 ounces)
Total Fat (grams)	53	73	93
Total Added Sugars (teaspoons)	6	12	18

**The lower number of servings (with recommended limits on fat and calories) applies to sedentary women. The middle number of servings applies to sendentary men. The highest level can also apply to very active women.*
***Women who are pregnant or breastfeeding, teenagers, and young adults to age 24 need 3 servings.*

How Many Servings Do You Need Each Day?

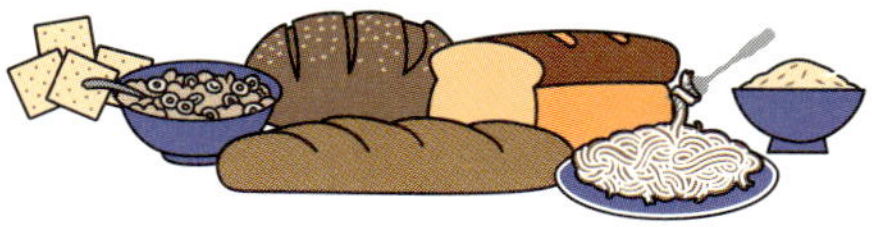

6 TO 11 SERVINGS FROM BREAD, CEREAL, RICE AND PASTA GROUP.

Eat products made from a variety of whole grains, such as wheat, rice, oats, corn, and barley. Select several servings of whole grain breads and cereals daily. Prepare and serve grain products with little or no fats and sugars. This group supplies the foundation of your diet. That's why it is the base — the foundation — of the Food Guide Pyramid.

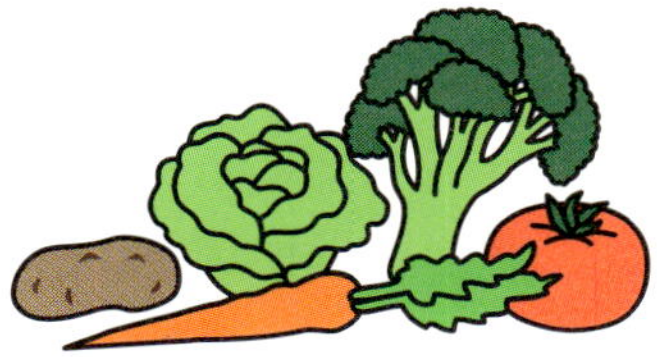

3 TO 5 SERVINGS FROM THE VEGETABLE GROUP.

This group includes dark green leafy vegetables such as spinach and broccoli; deep-yellow vegetables such as carrots and sweet potatoes; starchy vegetables such as potatoes and corn; dry beans, peas, and lentils; tomatoes, lettuce, onions, green beans, etc. These provide important vitamins such as Vitamin A, C, and folate, as well as minerals, including iron and magnesium. Prepare and serve vegetables with little or no fats.

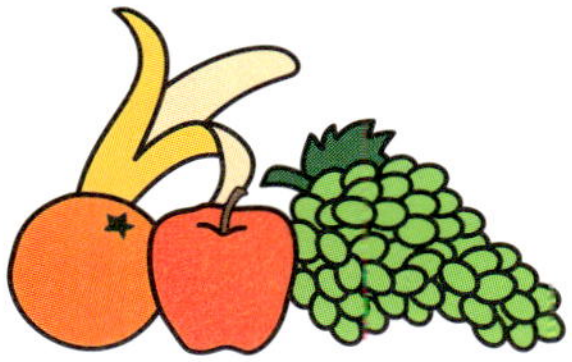

2 TO 4 SERVINGS FROM THE FRUIT GROUP.

This group includes fresh fruits, fruit juices and frozen, canned or dried fruit. Try to eat whole fruit often — not just fruit juices. Eat fruit as desserts or snacks. Have citrus fruit regularly; melons and berries, too. When counting juices, count only those that contain 100% fruit juice — punches, ades and most fruit "drinks" contain only a little fruit juice, and lots of sugar.

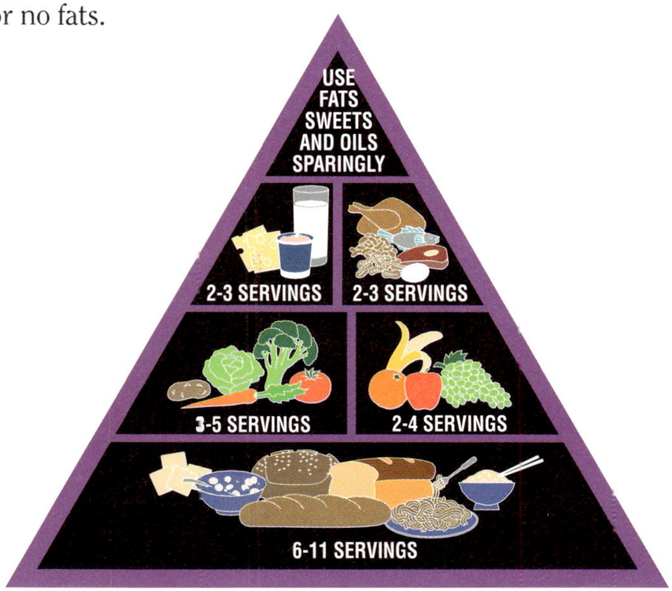

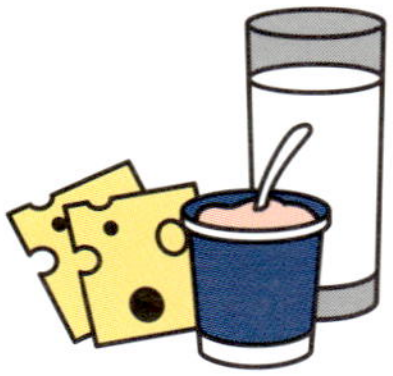

2 TO 3 SERVINGS FROM THE MILK, YOGURT AND CHEESE GROUP.

Teenagers and pregnant and breastfeeding women need three servings. These foods provide protein, calcium, as well as other minerals, and vitamins. This group includes not only milk, but cheese, cottage cheese, yogurt, even ice cream. However, it is best to choose lowfat milk and dairy products, such as skim or 1% milk, nonfat yogurt, lowfat ice cream, and part-skim or lowfat cheeses.

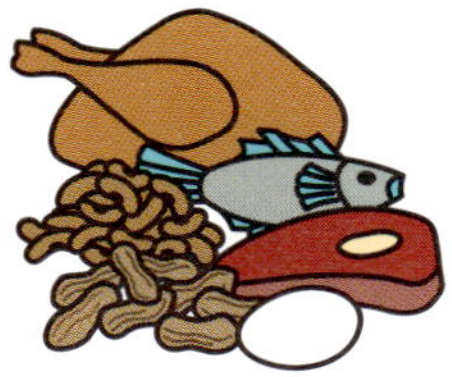

2 TO 3 SERVINGS FROM THE MEAT, POULTRY, FISH, DRY BEANS, EGGS AND NUTS GROUP.

This group provides protein, B vitamins, iron and zinc. Choose lean meats, such as beef round, beef loin; pork tenderloin, center loin; ham; veal, all cuts except ground; leg of lamb, loin, fore shank; chicken and turkey, both light and dark meat, without the skin; all kinds of fish. Vegetarian sources of protein, such as cooked dry beans, supply the same nutrients as do animal sources, and can substitute for part or all of the servings in this group.

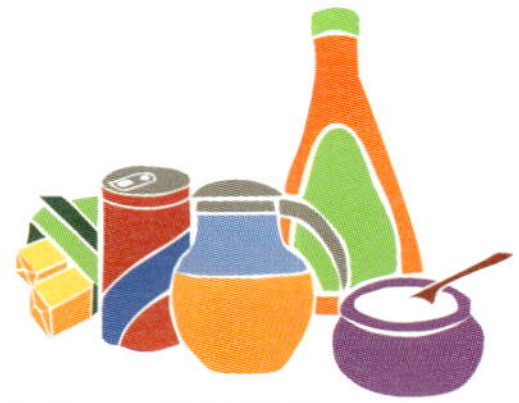

FATS, OILS AND SWEETS.

These foods supply calories, but few nutrients our bodies need. So it makes sense to be moderate in how much we eat. A little bit of added sugars and fats can make meals palatable, but it's important not to consume too much. Go easy on butter, margarine, gravy, salad dressing, sugar, jelly, sweet desserts, and soft drinks.

That's it. The Food Guide Pyramid allows plenty of flexibility. You can be a beef lover; you can be a vegetarian. Whatever your food preferences, the trick is to find the right balance that allows you to enjoy all the foods you love, in the right proportion.

It doesn't mean that every food, or even every meal, has to be low in fat. The goal is to find a balance you can live with, over several days. If you eat a big meal, with plenty of fat, one night, choose lower fat foods the next meal, or next day. If you find balance over several days, you'll do fine.

So will your children.

The Dietary Guidelines for Americans

THE DIETARY GUIDELINES are designed to help Americans choose diets that will meet nutrient requirements, promote health, support active lives, and reduce chronic disease risks. If you have a disease, such as heart disease or diabetes, you may need to follow a special diet under the supervision of a doctor. If your children are under the age of 2, they have special nutritional needs — for example, they should get breast milk or formula for the first year, and after that, whole milk rather than skim milk. If you have an infant, ask your pediatrician about what you should be feeding.

For every child age 2 and over, and every adult who is basically healthy, however, the 1995 Dietary Guidelines for Americans apply. It starts with the pleasure of good food. "Eating is one of life's greatest pleasures," reads the Guidelines. Whatever your ethnic, racial, or religious background, you can eat a diet consistent with the Dietary Guidelines. There are many different and pleasurable ways to combine foods to make healthful diets. Here are the basic principles:

EAT A VARIETY OF FOODS.
The Food Guide Pyramid illustrates the importance of balance among food groups in a daily eating pattern. Most of the daily servings of food should be selected from the food groups that are the largest in the picture and closest to the base of the pyramid.

BALANCE THE FOOD YOU EAT WITH PHYSICAL ACTIVITY — MAINTAIN OR IMPROVE YOUR WEIGHT.
If you are overweight, try to lose weight, or, at least try not to gain more weight. To burn more calories, become more physically active. Walk; use stairs; try to do 30 minutes a day on most days of moderate physical activity. Encourage your children to limit television watching, and, instead, play actively, in a safe environment. If your child is overweight, don't restrict calories, unless under supervision by a health professional. Instead, encourage healthful eating habits and more exercise.

CHOOSE A DIET WITH PLENTY OF GRAIN PRODUCTS, VEGETABLES, AND FRUITS.
Grain products, vegetables, and fruits are key parts of a varied diet; most of your calories should come from them. They provide vitamins, minerals, complex carbohydrates (starch and dietary fiber), and other substances important for good health. Eat products from a variety of whole grains, such as wheat, rice, oats, corn and barley. They are also generally low in fat, depending on how they are prepared and what is added to them at the table.

CHOOSE A DIET LOW IN FAT, SATURATED FAT AND CHOLESTEROL.
Saturated fat raises blood cholesterol. This increases the risk for heart disease. Saturated fats come mostly from meat, milk and dairy products, as well as many bakery products. So choose lower fat versions of these foods.

CHOOSE A DIET MODERATE IN SUGARS.

Sugar does not cause hyperactivity in children. But it often adds calories without nourishment. Avoid excessive snacking, especially on fatty, sugary foods.

CHOOSE A DIET MODERATE IN SALT AND SODIUM.

These come mainly from processed and prepared foods. Choose low sodium or reduced sodium versions of processed foods. Too much sodium may increase the risk of high blood pressure. In household measures, one level teaspoon of salt provides about 2,300 milligrams of sodium. Most people consume more than this amount. Consuming more fruits and vegetables also increases potassium intakes which may help to reduce blood pressure.

IF YOU DRINK ALCOHOLIC BEVERAGES, DO SO IN MODERATION.

Alcoholic beverages supply calories, but few or no nutrients. The alcohol in these beverages has effects that are harmful when consumed in excess. For some adults, moderate drinking — one drink a day for a woman, two for a man — may lower the risk of heart disease. (A drink is a 12 ounce beer, five ounces of wine, 1 ounces of 80 proof distilled spirits). But some people shouldn't drink at all: women who are pregnant or trying to get pregnant, anyone planning to drive soon, people taking certain medications, anyone who can't drink moderately — such as a recovering alcoholic. Children and adolescents should not drink at all.

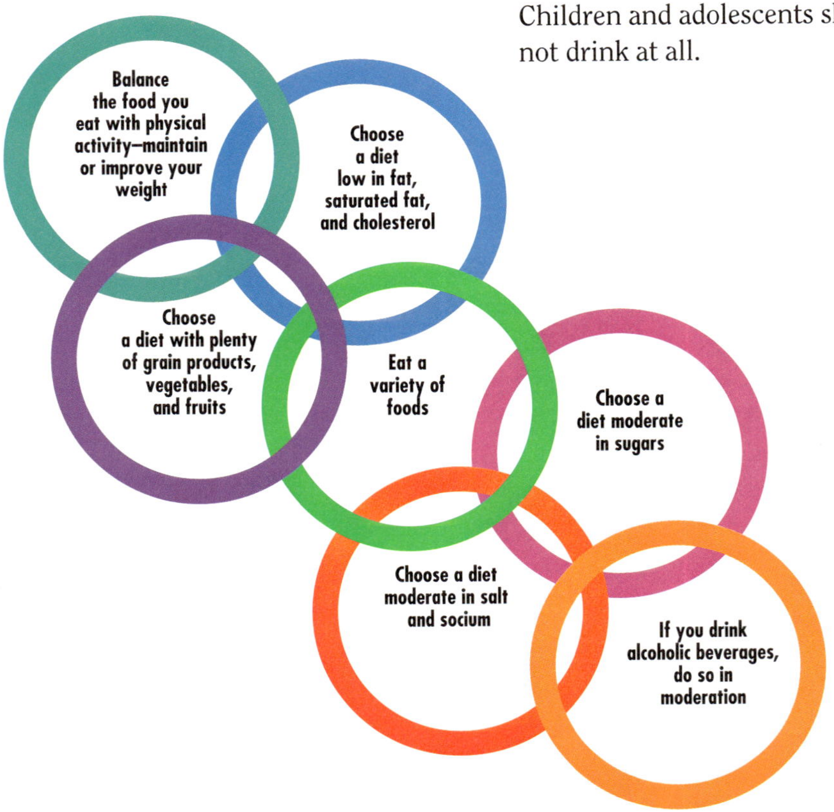

Making Healthful Food Choices

Easy Ways to Cut Fat

AT THE STORE

- Choose lean cuts of meat, such as beef round, loin, sirloin, pork loin chops, and roasts. All cuts with the name "loin" or "round" are lean.
- Select fish and poultry often; they are lower in saturated fat.
- Buy lowfat and nonfat versions of dairy products.
- Read the food labels and choose those foods that are lower in fat, saturated fat, and cholesterol.

AT THE TABLE

- Use less of all fats and oils, especially saturated fats such as butter, cream, sour cream, and cream cheese.
- Try nonfat salad dressings.
- As a beverage, gradually replace whole milk with 2% fat milk, then 1% fat or skim (nonfat) milk.

IN THE KITCHEN

- When cooking, replace saturated fats such as butter and lard with small amounts of polyunsaturated and monounsaturated fats in vegetable oils such as corn oil, soybean oil, olive oil, peanut oil, or canola oil.
- Broil, roast, bake, steam, or boil foods instead of frying them, or try stir-frying with just a little fat.
- Trim all visible fat from meats before cooking and remove the skin from poultry.
- Spoon off fat from meat dishes after they are cooked, and cooled.
- Use skim milk or lowfat milk when making "cream" sauces, soups, or puddings.
- Substitute lowfat yogurt or whipped lowfat cottage cheese for sour cream and mayonnaise in dips and dressings.
- Substitute two egg whites for each whole egg in recipes for most quick breads, cookies, and cakes. (The cholesterol and fat are in the yolk, not in the white.)
- Try lemon juice, herbs, or spices to season foods instead of butter or margarine.

Healthy Hints for Baking and Cooking

FOR...	USE...
1 whole egg	2 egg whites, or 1/4 cup cholesterol-free egg substitutes
Whole milk	Skim or lowfat milk
Sugar	Can be reduced to: 1/2 cup of sugar per cup of flour in cakes 1 tablespoon of sugar per cup of flour in yeast breads **Hint:** when reducing sugar, add more flavoring, such as vanilla
Baking chocolate, 1 oz.	3 tablespoons of cocoa (if fat is needed, use 1 tablespoon or less of oil)
Fat (vegetable oil, margarine, or butter)	Minimum for muffins and quick breads is 1 to 2 tablespoons of fat per cup of flour Minimum for cakes is 2 tablespoons of fat per cup of flour **Hint:** soft drop cookies generally contain less fat than rolled cookies
Sodium	Can be reduced to: 1/4 teaspoon of salt per cup of flour in yeast breads; half the amount of salt called for in other baked products 1-1/4 teaspoons of baking powder per cup of flour in muffins, biscuits, waffles 1 teaspoon of baking powder per cup of flour in cakes
Sour cream	Nonfat or lowfat sour cream or yogurt
Butter	Margarine or vegetable oil (total fat will be the same, but saturated fat and cholesterol will be reduced)
Cake flour (1 cup)	All-purpose flour (1 cup minus 2 tablespoons)
Solid shortening	Margarine or vegetable oil (If oil, use slightly less)
Vegetable oil (1/2 cup)	Applesauce (1/2 cup)
Shortening (l cup)	Shortening 1/2 cup and Applesauce 1/2 cup

Healthy Hints for Baking and Cooking

FOR...	USE...
Mayonnaise	Reduced-fat mayonnaise, nonfat, or plain yogurt
Heavy cream	Half and half, evaporated skim milk, fluid milk
Cheddar cheese	Mozzarella, part-skim, or low fat cheddar cheese
Cream cheese	Lowfat cream cheese, or fat-free cream cheese
Ricotta cheese	1% cottage cheese or skim milk ricotta cheese
Evaporated milk	Evaporated skim milk
Sweetened condensed milk	Low-fat sweetened condensed milk
Oil or margarine for frying	Vegetable spray
Deep-fat frying	Spray with vegetable oil and bake instead
Regular hamburger meat, spare ribs, prime cuts of meat, sausage	Lean, trimmed cuts of meat such as extra-lean hamburger, sirloin, or beef round; all fish and and shellfish; pork loin; veal; select or choice cuts of meat

FOR...	USE...
Bacon	Lean Canadian bacon
Salami, bologna, hot dogs, or liverwurst	Deli turkey breast, skinless chicken, lean roast beef, or boiled ham (trimmed), lower fat versions of hotdogs, such as turkey
Fried chicken or fried fish	Baked or broiled skinless chicken, fish, or turkey
Sausage, ground beef	Lean ground turkey or chicken, drained
Bread crumbs with butter	Cereal, crushed
Frosted cakes, cookies	Angel food cake, fat-free cake and cookies, graham crackers, and vanilla wafers
Doughnuts	Bagels, toast, english muffins
Buttered toast	Toast with jelly or preserves
Icing on cake	Dust with powdered sugar

Modifying Your Home Recipes

Any recipe, even your old favorites, can be modified to make them more healthful for your family. The recipes in this collection may give you ideas for modifying the recipes you're already using - by adding or substituting new ingredients, for example, and changing your cooking techniques.

When you decide to modify a recipe, start by making a small number of portions.

1. Change only one ingredient at a time. Keep other ingredients the same as in the original recipe.
2. Write down a clear description of foods substituted in exact amounts.
3. If increasing or decreasing an ingredient, do so in small amounts: 1/4 to 1/2 of the amount called for in the original recipe.
4. Follow directions closely and record any changes you may make.
5. Do not make further changes or a larger size recipe until the first change has produced an appetizing and good tasting product.

Once you have successfully prepared the recipe you modified, try the recipe again in a larger portion. It should work!

Try it out on your family. Evaluate the product for appearance, texture, flavor and overall acceptance.

Congratulations!

You've just modified your favorite recipe to make it healthful and tasty! Keep a record of your new recipe!

Note: The original recipe called for 1/2 cup of vegetable oil and 3 whole eggs. You can modify the recipe by lowering the fat to 1/4 cup of vegetable oil, or substitute with a 1/4 cup of applesauce. You can also use 2 eggs, or 4 egg whites, or 1/2 cup of cholesterol-free egg substitute to lower fat.

Easy Cake Delight

Cooking Time: 35 minutes Serves: 24

- 1 box of cake mix (chocolate, lemon, or any flavor)
- *¼ cup applesauce (or ¼ cup vegetable oil)*
- *2 eggs (or 4 egg whites or ½ cup cholesterol-free egg substitute)*
- 1¼ cup water
- 1 box instant pudding (chocolate, lemon, or any flavor)

1. **Spray** 9" x 13" pan with vegetable spray.
2. **Mix** together the above ingredients. Beat until fluffy.
3. **Bake** at 350°F for 35 minutes.

Nutrients per serving
1 slice

Calories	117	Saturated Fat	0.5 g	Iron	0.4 mg
Protein	1 g	Cholesterol	18 mg	Calcium	32 mg
Carbohydrate	21 g	Vitamin A	8 RE	Sodium	208 mg
Total Fat	2.9 g	Vitamin C	0 mg	Dietary Fiber	0 g

Reading the Food Label

The new food label makes it easier than ever to choose healthy foods quickly. The more you use it, the easier it is to use. Here are a few tips to introduce you to the new food label.

TAKE A MINUTE AND CHECK OUT THE "NUTRITION FACTS" PANEL ON NEW LABELS.

Notice it's easier to see the nutrients, many of which are new on labels: saturated fat, cholesterol, dietary fiber and sugars. All nutrients will be listed in the same order so they're easy to find and compare.

THINK ABOUT YOUR REASONS FOR USING THE NEW LABEL.

Are you concerned about limiting fat or sodium in your diet?

Do you want to increase the amount of fiber and calcium?

You may want to pick only one or two things to look at. Remember, you do not need to know everything on the label. Focus on what is most important to you.

LOOK AT THE PERCENT DAILY VALUE COLUMN ON THE RIGHT OF THE "NUTRITION FACTS" PANEL.

It's also new and very important: it tells you if a number is high (or low) in a nutrient like fat, cholesterol, or sodium. If a serving provides 5% or less of the Daily Value, it is low in that nutrient and represents a minor part of your diet. So you can look at a single food to see what nutrients it is high or low in, or you can use this column to compare two different foods.

BE SURE TO COMPARE HOW MUCH YOU ACTUALLY EAT WITH THE SIZE OF THE SERVING ON THE PACKAGE.

Remember, the number of calories and the nutrient amounts are based on the serving size shown on the label. **You may eat more or less.** If you eat two servings, you'll need to double the percent Daily Value for all the nutrients listed.

LOOK FOR CLAIMS ON THE FRONT OF PACKAGES; THEY MEAN WHAT THEY SAY.

Check the percent Daily Value column on the "Nutrition Fact" panel to compare claims like "lite" and "low fat".

The New Food Label: Check it Out!

Nutrition Facts

Serving Size 1/2 cup (114g)
Servings Per Container 4

Amount Per Serving

Calories 100 Calories from Fat 30

	% Daily Value*
Total Fat 3g	**5%**
Saturated Fat 0g	**0%**
Cholesterol 30mg	**10%**
Sodium 660mg	**28%**
Total Carbohydrate 13g	**4%**
Dietary Fiber 3g	**12%**
Sugars 5g	
Protein 5g	

Vitamin A 4% • Vitamin C 2%
Calcium 15% • Iron 4%

Percent Daily Values are based on a 2,000 calorie diet. Your daily values may be higher or lower depending on your calorie needs:

	Calories:	2,000	2,500
Total Fat	Less than	65g	80g
* Sat Fat	Less than	20g	25g
Cholesterol	Less than	300mg	300mg
Sodium	Less than	2,400mg	2,400mg
Total Carbohydrate		300g	375g
Dietary Fiber		25g	30g

Calories per gram:
Fat 9 • Carbohydrate 4 • Protein 4

Finding Nutrition Information

Contact a local community nutritionist, public health nutritionist, extension agent or specialist, home economist, or local dietitian from a hospital or university, dietetic association, diabetes association, heart association, or cancer society. For other health professionals, contact your local or state health department.

LOCAL COOPERATIVE EXTENSION SERVICE OFFICES

Cooperative Extension Service offices are a source of nutrition education resources, programs, and Team Nutrition related youth, family, and community activities. The local offices are usually in courthouses, post offices, or other government buildings. Telephone numbers are usually listed in the telephone directory under county/city government and often the listing includes the name of the land-grant university.

STATE EXTENSION CONTACTS FOR USDA'S TEAM NUTRITION

Cooperative Extension Service state offices are located on the campuses of land-grant universities. Below is a list of Cooperative Extension faculty who are a source of research-based nutrition information including Team Nutrition.

NATIONAL OFFICE

The national office is located in the U.S. Department of Agriculture, Washington, DC.

Cooperative State Research, Education and Extension Service (CSREES)
Families, 4-H, and Nutrition
CSREES, USDA
Stop 2225
1400 Independence Avenue, SW
Washington, DC 20250-2225
Tel: (202) 720-2908
Fax: (202) 690-2469

or contact via Email:
CSREES@reeusda.gov
or on the CSREES Home Page
on the World Wide Web at
http://www.reeusda.gov

State Extension Contacts for USDA's Team Nutrition

AMERICAN SAMOA
Dr. Carol S. Whitaker
State Coordinator
Family & Consumer Science
Land Grant Program, American Samoa Community College
P.O. Box 5319
Pago Pago, AS 96799
Tel: (684) 699-1394
Fax: (684) 699-4595
Email: wit@elele.peacesat.hawaii.edu

ALABAMA
Dr. Eunice A. Bonsi
Nutrition Educator/Family Life Specialist
Tuskegee University
Kellogg Conference Center
Extension/Continuing Education Office
Tuskegee, AL 36088
Tel: (334) 727-8816
Fax: (334) 724-4199
Email: ebonsi@acd.tusk.edu

Dr. Barbara Struepler
Nutrition Specialist
207 Duncan Hall
Auburn University, AL 36849
Tel: (334) 844-2217
Fax: (334) 884-5354
Email: bstruemp@acenet.auburn.edu

ALASKA
Dr. Bret Luick
Food & Nutrition Specialist
Alaska Cooperative Extension
University of Alaska-Fairbanks
P.O. Box 756180
Fairbanks, AK 99775-6180
Tel: (907) 474-6338
Fax: (907) 474-7439
Email: ffbrl@aurora.alaska.edu

ARIZONA
Dr. Linda Houtkooper
Nutrition Specialist
University of Arizona
Department of Nutritional Sciences
Room 312, FCR Building
P.O. Box 210033
Tucson, AZ 85721-0033
Tel: (520) 621-7126
Fax: (520) 621-9445
Email: houtkoop@ag.arizona.edu

ARKANSAS
Dr. Irene K. Lee
Ext. Family/Child Development Spec.
University of Arkansas/Pine Bluff
1890 Extension Program
Box 4966
Pine Bluff, AR 71601
Tel: (501) 543-8530
Fax: (501) 543-8166

Dr. Rosemary Rodibaugh
Extension Nutrition Specialist
University of Arkansas, CES
P.O. Box 391, 2301 South University Avenue
Little Rock, AR 72204
Tel: (501) 671-2111
Fax: (501) 671-2251
Email: rrodibaugh@uaex.edu

CALIFORNIA
Dr. Marilyn Townsend
Nutrition Specialist
Department of Nutrition
University of California - Davis
1145 Meyer Hall
Davis, CA 95616
Tel: (916) 754-9222
Fax: (916) 752-7588
Email: mstownsend@ucdavis.edu

COLORADO
Dr. Jennifer Anderson
Extension Nutrition Specialist
Colorado State University
200-A Gifford Hall
Fort Collins, CO 80523
Tel: (970) 491-7334
Fax: (970) 491-7252
Email: jela@lamar.colostate.edu

CONNECTICUT
Dr. Colleen Thompson
University of Connecticut-CES
Dept. of Nutrition Science
3624 Horsebarn Road - U17
Storrs, CT 06269-4017
Tel: (860) 486-1784
Fax: (860) 486-3674
Email: cthompson@canr1.cag.uconn.edu

DELAWARE
Dr. Sue Snider
Extension Specialist
Food and Nutrition
University of Delaware
123 Townsend Hall
Newark, DE 19717-1303
Tel: (302) 831-2509
Fax: (302) 831-3651
Email: sue.snider@mvs.udel.edu

DISTRICT OF COLUMBIA
Dr. Lillie Monroe-Lord
Extension Specialist
University of the District of Columbia, CES
901 Newton Street, N.E., Room 302
Washington, DC 20017
Tel: (202) 274-6904/6900
Fax: (202 274-6930/6980
Email: jhazel@esusda.gov

Extension Contacts — continued

FLORIDA

Ms. Glenda L. Warren
Nutrition-EFNEP-Specialist
3031-B McCarty Hall
University of Florida
P.O. Box 110310
Gainesville, FL 32611-0310
Tel: (352) 392-0404
Fax: (352) 392-8196
Email: glw@gnv.ifas.ufl.eduAssoc. Professor

Dr. Mabel Edlow
Extension Specialist
Florida A&M University
215 Perry Paige Building
Tallahassee, FL 32307
Tel: (904) 561-2095
Fax: (904) 561-2151
Email: medlow@ns1.famu.edu

GEORGIA

Dr. Elizabeth Andress
Extension Leader/Food, Nutrition & Health
CES Family & Consumer Sciences
208 Hoke Smith Annex
The University of Georgia
Athens, GA 30602-4356
Tel: (706) 542-3773
Fax: (706) 542-1979
Email: eandress@uga.cc.uga.edu

Dr. Carol A. Johnson
Leader/Home Economics & Family Dev.
Fort Valley State College
1890 Extension Programs
P.O. Box 4061
Fort Valley, GA 31030-3298
Tel: (912) 825-6298
Fax: (912) 825-6299
Email: cjohnson@fvs3.fvsc.peachnet.edu

GUAM

Dr. Erlinda L. Demeterio
Chair, Consumer & Family Sciences Unit, CES
College of Agriculture & Life Sciences
University of Guam
UOG Station
Mangilao, GU 96923
Tel: (671) 735-2000/9
Fax: (671) 734-6842
Email: demeteri@uog.edu

HAWAII

Dr. Patricia Britten
Food & Nutrition Specialist
Department of Food Science & Human Nutrition
1800 East-West Road, Pope 120A
Honolulu, HI 96822
Tel: (808) 956-6457
Fax: (808) 956-3842
Email: trish@hawaii.edu

IDAHO

Linda Gossett
Extension Specialist
University of Idaho
800 Park Blvd., Suite 200
Boise, ID 83714
Tel: (208) 345-5812
Fax: (208) 375-8715
Email: lgossett@uidaho.edu

ILLINOIS

Dr. Robin A. Orr
University of Illinois/CES
520C Bevier Hall
905 South Goodwin Avenue
Urbana, IL 61801
Tel: (217) 244-2855
Fax: (217) 244-2861
Email: orrr@idea.ag.uiuc.edu

INDIANA

Dr. Bill Evers
Ext. Spec/Foods & Nutrition
Purdue University
G-1g Stone Hall
West Lafayette, IN 47907
Tel: (317) 765-8546
Fax: (317) 765-0674
Email: eversb@cfs.purdue.edu

IOWA

Ms. Elisabeth A. Schafer
Professor, Food Science/Human Nutrition
1127 Human Nutrition Science Building
Iowa State University
1105 LeBaron Hall
Ames, IA 50011
Tel: (515) 294-1359
Fax: (515) 294-6193
Email: eschafer@iastate.edu

KANSAS

Dr. Paula Peters
Developmental Nutrition Specialist
Kansas State University, CES
Justin Hall
Manhattan, KS 66506-1407
Tel: (913) 532-1666
Fax: (913) 532-3132
Email: peters@humec.ksu.edu

KENTUCKY

Dr. Janet Kurzynske
Extension Food & Nutrition Specialist
Rm. 234, Scovell Hall
University of Kentucky
Lexington, KY 40546-0064
Tel: (606) 257-1812
Fax: (606) 257-7792
Email: jkurzyns@ca.uky.edu

Mary J. Fant
State Specialist - Children and Youth
Family and Management
Kentucky State University CES
Box 196
Frankfort, KY 40601
Tel: (502) 227-6955
Fax: (502) 227-5933
Email: mfant@ca.uky.edu

LOUISIANA

Donna Montgomery, R.D.
Nutrition Specialist
Lousiana State University CES
P.O. Box 25100
Baton Rouge, LA 70894-5100
Tel: (504) 388-3329
Fax: (504) 388-2478
Email: xthome@lsuvm.sncc.lsu.edu

Dr. Gina Eubanks
Associate Specialists, CES
Southern University and A&M College
P.O. Box 10010
Baton Rouge, LA 70813
Tel: (504) 771-2242
Fax: (504) 771-2861
Email: gina3902@aol.com

MAINE

Nellie G. Hedstrom, R.D.
Nutrition Specialist Coop. Exr.
5717 Corbett Hall, Room 300
University of Maine
Orono, ME 04469-5717
Tel: (207) 581-3110
Fax: (207) 581-3212
Email: nellieh@umce.umext.maine.edu

MARIANAS

Ms. Floria P. James
Home Economist, Agriculture & Life Sciences
Northern Marianas College
P.O. Box 1250
Saipan, MP 96950
Tel: (670) 234-9025
Fax: (670) 234-0054

MARYLAND

Dr. Maria M. deColon
EFNEP Coordinator
University of Maryland, CES
2309 Computer Science Bldg.
College Park, MD 20742-2451
Tel: (301) 405-1016
Fax: (301) 314-9015
Email: md15@umail.umd.edu

Gayle Mason-Jenkins
Extension Specialist - Home Ec.
University of Maryland - Eastern Shore
Eastern Shore, Backbone Road
Princess Anne, MD 21853
Tel: (410) 651- 1212
Fax: (410) 651- 6207
Email: gjenkins@umes-bird.umd.edu

MASSACHUSETTS

Dr. Nancy Cohen
Nutrition Education Specialist
Box 31420
201 Chenoworth Lab
University of Massachusetts
Amherst, MA 01003-1430
Tel: (413) 545-0740
Fax: (413) 545-1074
Email: cohen@nutrition.umass.edu

MICHIGAN

Pat Hammerschmidt
Program Leader
Children, Youth and Family
Michigan State University Extension
103 Human Ecology Building
East Lansing, MI 48824-1030
Tel: (517) 355-6586
Fax: (517) 353-6343
Email: hammersc@msuces.canr.msu.edu

MINNESOTA

Mr. Craig Hassell
Extension Nutritionist
University of Minnesota
225 Food Science and Nutrition Bldg.
1334 Eckles Avenue
St. Paul, MN 55108
Tel: (612) 624-2703
Fax: (612) 625-6227
Email: chassel@mes.umn.edu

MISSISSIPPI

Dr. Barbara P. McLaurin
Extension Human Nutrition Specialist
P.O. Box 9745
Mississippi State, MS 39762
Tel: (601) 325-3080
Fax: (601) 325-8407
Email: barbaram@mces.msstate.edu

Mrs. Deborah Caples-Davis
Nutritionist
Alcorn Extension Service
P.O. Box 61 North
Port Gibson, MS 39150
Tel: (601) 437-3052
Fax: (601) 437-3051

MISSOURI

Ms. Ann Cohen
Assoc. State Extension Specialist
Food Science & Human Nutrition
University of Missouri-Columbia
301 Gwynn Hall
Columbia, MO 65211
Tel: (573) 882-2435
Fax: (573) 884-5449
Email: cohena@ext.missouri.edu

MONTANA

Ms. Phyllis Dennee
Nutrition Education Specialist
101 Rommney
Montana State University
Bozeman, MT 59717
Tel: (406) 994-4581
Fax: (406) 994-6314
Email: ihdpd@msu.oscs.montana.edu

NEBRASKA

Dr. Linda Boeckner
Ext. Nutrition Specialist
NE Research and Extension Center
Box 111
Concord, NE 68728
Tel: (402) 584-2261
Fax: (402) 584-2859
Email: nerc010@unlvm.unl.edu

NEVADA

Dr. Jamie Benedict
Extension Specialist
Department of Nutrition
University of Nevada-Reno
Reno, NV 89557
Tel: (702) 784-6445
Fax: (702) 784-6449
Email: benedict@scs.unr.edu

NEW HAMPSHIRE

Ms. Valerie A. Long
Extension Specialist, Food & Nutrition
220 Kendall Hall, 129 Main Street
University of New Hampshire
Durham, NH 03824
Tel: (603) 862-2465
Fax: (603) 862-3758
Email: valerie.long@unh.edu

Extension Contacts — continued

NEW JERSEY
Dr. Mary Jane Willis
Specialist in Nutrition
Rutgers Cooperative Extension
134 Thompson Hall, P.O. Box 231
New Brunswick, NJ 08903-0231
Tel: (908) 932-9853
Fax: (908) 932-6837
Email: keenan@aesop.rutgers.edu

NEW MEXICO
Ms. Martha Archuleta, R.D.
Extension Food & Nutrition Specialist
New Mexico State University
Box 3AE
Las Cruces, NM 88003
Tel: (505) 646-3516
Fax: (505) 646-5263
Email: maarchul@nmsu.edu

NEW YORK
Christina Stark, R.D.
Extension Nutrition Specialist
Div. of Nutritional Sciences
MVR Hall, Cornell University
Ithaca, NY 14853
Tel: (607) 255-2141
Fax: (607) 255-0027
Email: cms11@Cornell.edu

NORTH CAROLINA
Dr. Wilda Wade
Foods & Nutrition Specialist/Dietetics Director
P.O. Box 21928
North Carolina A&T State Univ.
Greensboro, NC 27420-1928
Tel: (910) 334-7660
Fax: (910) 334-7265
Email: wadew@rhema.ncat.edu

Dr. P. Carolyn Dunn
Food and Nutrition Specialist
North Carolina State Univ. - CES
Box 7605
Raleigh, NC 27695-7605
Tel: (919) 515-9142
Fax: (919) 515-3483
Email: pcdunn@amaroq.ces.ncsu.edu

NORTH DAKOTA
Dr. Julie Garden-Robinson
Foods & Nutrition Extension Specialist
219 Family Life Center, NDSU
Fargo, ND 58105-5016
Tel: (701) 231-7187
Fax: (701) 231-8568
Email: jgardenr@ndsuext.nodak.edu

OHIO
Dr. Alma Saddam
Nutrition Specialist
Ohio State University
1787 Neil Avenue
Columbus, OH 43210
Tel: (614) 292-5512
Fax: (614) 292-7536
Email: saddam.1@osu.edu

OKLAHOMA
Dr. Barbara Brown
Extension Food Specialist
Dept. of Nutritional Sciences
Oklahoma State University
309 Human Environmental Sciences
Stillwater, OK 74078-6111
Tel: (405) 744-6824
Fax: (405) 744-7113
Email: bbrown@okway.okstate.edu

Alice Delano Campbell
Extension Specialist
Langston University
101N Research Building
P.O. Box 730
Langston, OK 73050
Tel: (405) 466-3836
Fax: (405) 466-3138
Email: ext1890@mvs.ucc.okstate.edu

OREGON
Dr. Carolyn Raab
Ext. Food & Nutrition Specialist
Oregon State University
161 Milam Hall
Corvallis, OR 97331-5106
Tel: (541) 737-1019
Fax: (541) 737-0999
Email: raabc@ccmail.orst.edu

PENNSYLVANIA
Dr. Jan Scholl
Assoc. Professor, Ext. Edu.
323 Ag. Admin. Building
Penn. State University
University Park, PA 16802
Tel: (814) 863-7869
Fax: (814) 863-4753
Email: jan_scholl@agcs.cas.psu.edu

PUERTO RICO
Dr. Ann Macpherson de Sanchez
Associate Specialist, Ag Ext Service
P.O. Box 5000 - College Station
University of Puerto Rico - Mayaguez Campus
Mayaguez, PR 00680
Tel: (787) 832-4040 Ext. 3348
Fax: (787) 265-4130
Email:
A_MACPHERSON@SEAM.UPR.CLU.EDU

RHODE ISLAND
Ms. Linda Sebelia
Director, EFNEP Program
Dept. of Food Science & Nutrition
URI Providence Center
80 Washington Street
Providence, RI 02903
Tel: (401) 277-5278
Fax: (401) 277-5319
Email: sebelia@uriacc.uri.edu

SOUTH CAROLINA
Ms. Margaret E. Johnson
Associate Administrator, 1890 Extension
South Carolina State University
300 College Street, N.E.
P.O. Box 7336
Orangeburg, SC 29117
Tel: (803) 536-8465
Fax: (803) 536-7102
Email: mjhnsn@clemson.edu

Dr. Rose J. Davis,
Extension Nutrition Specialist
Pee Dee Research & Education Center
Clemson University
2200 Pocket Road
Florence, SC 29506-9706
Tel: (803) 669-1912 Ext. 232
Fax: (803) 661-5676
Email: rdavis@clemson.edu

SOUTH DAKOTA
Carol Pitts, R.D.
Extension Food & Nutrition Specialist
South Dakota State Univ.
NHE 239, Box 2275-A
Brookings, SD 57007
Tel: (605) 688-6233
Fax: (605) 688-6360
Email: pittsc@mg.sdstate.edu

TENNESSEE
Betty P. Greer
Asst. Professor
Home Economics/Food, Nutrition and Health
University of Tennessee
P.O. Box 1071
Knoxville, TN 37901-1071
Tel: (423) 974-8746
Fax: (423) 974-7448
Email: bgreer@utk.edu

TEXAS
Dr. Katheleen Ladewig
Program Leader for Foods & Nutrition
Texas A&M University, CES
Human Nutrition Section
353 Kleberg Center
College Station, TX 77843-2471
Tel: (409) 845-6379
Fax: (409) 847-8741
Email: k-ladewig@tamu.edu

Dr. Linda Williams-Willis
Administrator, 1890 Programs
Prairie View A&M University
P.O. Box 3059
Prairie View, TX 77446
Tel: (409) 857-3812
Fax: (409) 857-2637
Email: lw-willis@tamu.edu

UTAH
Dr. Georgia C. Lauritzen
Associate Professor & EFNEP Director
Nutrition & Food Sciences Department
Utah State University
Logan, UT 84322-8749
Tel: (801) 797-3464
Fax: (801) 797-2379
Email: georgial@ext.usu.edu

VERMONT
Ms. Linda Lyons
EFNEP Coordinator
University of Vermont
Terrill Hall
Burlington, VT 05405-0148
Tel: (802) 656-0669
Fax: (802) 656-0407
Email: lyons@zoo.uvm.edu

VIRGIN ISLANDS
Mrs. Josephine Petersen-Springer
Program Leader/Home Economics
University of the Virgin Islands-CES
RR#2, Box 10,000 Kingshill
St. Croix, VI 00850
Tel: (809) 692-4096
Fax: (809) 692-4085

VIRGINIA
Dr. Ann Hertzler
Extension Specialist
Foods and Nutrition
338 Wallace Hall
Virginia Tech
Blacksburg, VA 24061-0430
Tel: (540) 231-4673
Fax: (540) 231-3916
Email: hertzler@vt.edu

WASHINGTON
Ms. Sue Butkus
Extension Nutrition Specialist
Washington State University
7612 Pioneer Way East
Puyallup, WA 98371-4998
Tel: (206) 840-4553
Fax: (206) 840-4671
Email: butkus@wsu.edu

WEST VIRGINIA
Dr. Guendoline Brown
Ext. Spec. - Nutrition & Health
West Virginia University, CES
605 Knapp Hall
P.O. Box 6031
Morgantown, WV 26506-6031
Tel: (304) 293-2694
Fax: (304) 293-7599
Email: brown@wvnvms.wvnet.edu

WISCONSIN
Dr. Susan Nitzke
Nutrition Specialist, Associate Professor
Nutritional Sciences, UW-Madison
1415 Linden Drive
275 Nutritional Sciences Building
Madison, WI 53706-1571
Tel: (608) 262-1692
Fax: (608) 262-5860
Email: nitzke@nutrisci.wisc.edu

WYOMING
Virginia Ann Romero, R.D.
Nutrition Specialist
University of Wyoming
P.O. Box 1929
Rock Springs, WY 82902
Tel: (307) 352-6775
Fax: (307) 352-6779
Email: vromero@wwcc.cc.wy.us

Regional USDA Team Nutrition Contacts

NORTHEAST REGION
Connecticut, Maine, Massachusetts, New Hampshire, New York, Rhode Island, Vermont

Charles DeJulius
USDA/FCS/NERO
10 Causeway Street, Room 501
Boston, Massachusetts 02222-1068
(617) 565-6418

MID-ATLANTIC REGION
Delaware, District of Columbia, Maryland, New Jersey, Pennsylvania, Puerto Rico, Virginia, Virgin Islands, West Virginia

Walt Haake
USDA/FCS/MARO
Mercer Corporate Park
300 Corporate Blvd.
Robbinsville, New Jersey 08691-1598
(609) 259-5091

SOUTHEAST REGION
Alabama, Florida, Georgia, Kentucky, Mississippi, North Carolina, South Carolina, Tennessee

Sara Harding
USDA/FCS/SERO
77 Forsyth Street, SW, Suite 112
Atlanta, Georgia 30303-3427
(404) 730-2588

MIDWEST REGION
Illinois, Indiana, Michigan, Minnesota, Ohio, Wisconsin

Lawrence Rudmann
USDA/FCS/MWRO
77 West Jackson Blvd., 20th Floor
Chicago, Illinois 60604-3507
(312) 353-1044

SOUTHWEST REGION
Arkansas, Louisiana, New Mexico, Oklahoma, Texas

Judy Barron
USDA/FCS/SWRO
1100 Commerce St., Rm 5-C-30
Dallas, Texas 75242
(214) 767-0256

MOUNTAIN PLAINS REGION
Colorado, Iowa, Kansas, Missouri, Montana, Nebraska, North Dakota, South Dakota, Utah, Wyoming

Darlene Sanchez
USDA/FCS/MPRO
1244 Speer Blvd., Suite 903
Denver, Colorado 80204
(303) 844-0355

WESTERN REGION
Alaska, Arizona, California, Hawaii, Idaho, Nevada, Oregon, Washington, Guam

Cordelia Morris
USDA/FCS/WRO
550 Kearny Street, Rm 400
San Francisco, California 94108-2518
(415) 705-1311

Looking for a Farmers' Market

FARMERS' MARKETS - LOOK FOR THE NEAREST ONE IN YOUR LOCAL COMMUNITY.

Most farmers' markets are sponsored by cities, chambers of commerce, farmer cooperatives and local not-for-profit organizations working to enhance the community and local agriculture. Typically, the markets are located on downtown public streets, squares, plazas and parking lots, in neighborhood parks, at shopping malls or at designated market facilities under open-air sheds.

Below is a sampling of local farmers' markets across the nation. (We have listed only two for each State). For those involved in planning and developing farmers' markets around the country or for a complete listing of all farmers' markets a new directory is available: 1996 National Farmers' Market Directory. For a copy, write to:

USDA/AMS/TMD/W&AM
P.O. Box 96456, Room 2642-South
Washington, D.C. 20090-6456
Phone: (202)720-8317

The Internet address of the directory is: http://www.usda.gov/ams/states.htm

LIST OF KEY FARMERS' MARKETS

ALABAMA

Jefferson County Truck Growers Association
414 West Finley Avenue
Birmingham, AL 35204
Contact: Danny Jones
(205) 251-8737
YEAR-ROUND

Montgomery State Farmers' Market
1655 Federal Drive
Montgomery, AL 36109
Contact: Benny Hitch
(205) 242-5350
YEAR-ROUND

ALASKA

Central Kenai Peninsula Farmers' Market
PO Box 988
Kenai, AK 99611
Contact: Leah Spaulding
(907) 283-3633
OPEN-AIR/SEASONAL

Saturday Farmers' Market
700 6th Avenue, Suite 206
Anchorage, AK 99501
Contact: Dave Harbour
(907) 276-8970
OPEN-AIR/SEASONAL

ARIZONA

Heritage Square Farmers' Market
7th & Monroe Streets
Phoenix, AZ 85034
Contact: Dee or John Logan
(602) 848-1234
YEAR-ROUND

Sun City-Campana Square Farmers' Market
98th Avenue & Bell Road
Sun City, AZ 85351
Contact: Dee or John Logan
(602) 848-1234
OPEN-AIR/SEASONAL

ARKANSAS

Downtown Farmers' Market
6th & Scott Streets
Little Rock, AR 72201
Contact: Christy Copeland
(501) 375-0121
OPEN-AIR/SEASONAL

Fayetteville Farmers' Market
The Square
Fayetteville, AR 72701
Contact: Sara Pollard
(501) 634-7122
OPEN-AIR/SEASONAL

CALIFORNIA

Los Angeles Adams & Vermont Farmers' Market
St. Agnes Catholic Church parking lot
Los Angeles, CA 90007
Contact: Roy Edwards
(213) 777-1755
YEAR-ROUND

San Francisco Heart of the City Farmers' Market
Market & 7th Streets
San Francisco, CA 94102
Contact: Christine Adams
(415) 558-9455
YEAR-ROUND

COLORADO

Denver Farmers' Market
17th & Market Street
Denver, CO 80202
Contact: Verne Batchelder
(303) 794-7768
OPEN-AIR/SEASONAL

Ft. Collins Farmers' Market
Mountain & Mason Streets
Ft. Collins, CO 80524
Contact: Kenneth Hall or Kathleen Mannix
(970) 493-1427
OPEN-AIR/SEASONAL

Farmers' Markets — continued

CONNECTICUT

Hartford/Park Street Farmers' Market
Park & Washington Streets
Hartford, CT 06112
Contact: Brian Kelliher
(860) 749-4186
OPEN-AIR/SEASONAL

New Haven Farmers' Market
Orange Street, Pitkin Plaza
New Haven, CT 06473
Contact: James Clouse, Sr.
(203) 272-2372
OPEN-AIR/SEASONAL

DELAWARE

Wilmington Farmers' Market
8th & Orange Streets
Wilmington, DE 19801
Contact: Beverly Zimmerman
(302) 571-9088
YEAR-ROUND

DISTRICT OF COLUMBIA

DC Open Air Farmers' Market
Oklahoma Avenue & Benning Road - RFK Stadium
Washington, DC 20002
Contact: Al Smith
(202) 728-2800
OPEN-AIR/SEASONAL

Eastern Market
7th & South Carolina Avenue SE
Washington, DC 20032
Contact: Al Smith
(202) 543-7293
YEAR-ROUND

FLORIDA

Fort Myers Farmers' Market
P. O. Box 187, 2744 Edison Avenue
Ft. Myers, FL 33916
Contact: Clad Brockett
(941) 332-6910
YEAR-ROUND

Gadsden County Farmers' Market
U.S. 90 West, Route 4, Box 1228-F
Quincy, FL 32351
Contact: Jim Warner
(904) 627-6484
YEAR-ROUND

GEORGIA

Atlanta State Farmers' Market
16 Forest Parkway
Forest Park, GA 30050
Contact: Mike Bonner
(404) 366-6910
YEAR-ROUND

Thomasville State Farmers' Market
502 Smith Avenue
Thomasville, GA 31792
Contact: Rex Gay
(912) 225-4072
YEAR-ROUND

IDAHO

Downtown Boise Farmers' Market
8th & Main Street
Boise, ID 83702
Contact: Helen Miller
(208) 336-0267
OPEN-AIR/SEASONAL

Twin Falls Farmers' Market
Saturday - 2318 Addison Avenue East
Every other Tuesday - Main & 2nd Street South
Twin Falls, ID 83301
Contact: Steve Tanguy
(208) 734-7134
OPEN-AIR/SEASONAL

ILLINOIS

Chicago Farmers' Market, Logan Square
63rd & Halsted
Chicago, IL 60602
Contact: Constance Buscemi
(312) 744-4006
OPEN-AIR SEASONAL

Springfield Farmers' Market
Downtown Square
Springfield, IL 62701
Contact: Paul Edwards
(217) 789-2255
OPEN-AIR/SEASONAL

INDIANA

Bloomington Community Farmers' Market
East 6th Street
Bloomington, IN 47408
Contact: Craig Brenner
(812) 331-6430
OPEN-AIR/SEASONAL

Lafayette Farmers' Market
5th Street between Main & Columbia Streets
Lafayette, IN 47901
Contact: Susan Smith
(317) 742-2313
OPEN-AIR/SEASONAL

IOWA

Davenport Association Farmers' Market
Gaines & Western Avenues on River Drive
Davenport, IA 52802
Contact: Ken Nelson
(319) 787-2429
OPEN-AIR/SEASONAL

Downtown Des Moines Farmers' Market
4th& Court Avenues
Des Moines, IA 50309
Contact: Toni Wilson
(515) 245-3880
OPEN-AIR/SEASONAL

KANSAS

Topeka Farmers' Market
10th & Topeka Boulevard
Topeka, KS 66612
Contact: Mary Fritts
(913) 234-9336
OPEN-AIR/SEASONAL

Wichita Farmers' Market
21st & Ridge
Wichita, KS 67202
Contact: Sandy Allen
(316) 796-1994
OPEN-AIR/SEASONAL

KENTUCKY

Lexington Farmers' Market
Vine Street
Lexington, KY 40507
Contact: Kate Kriegel
(502) 863-1517
OPEN-AIR/SEASONAL

Louisville Farmers' Market
Crescent Hill Methodist Church, Frankfort Avenue
Louisville, KY 40206
Contact: Maupin Cantrell
(502) 896-0396
OPEN-AIR/SEASONAL

LOUISIANA

Iberia Parish Farmers' Market
Sugar Cane Festival Building
New Iberia, LA 70562
Contact: Norris Grabert
(318) 369-4440
SEASONAL

Shreveport Farmers' Market
Parking lot of Expot Hall
Shreveport, LA 71101
Contact: Charles Lombardino
(318) 673-7700
SEASONAL

MAINE

Auburn Mall Farmers' Market
Porteous rear lot, Turner Street side
Auburn, ME 04210
Contact: Leo Tetreault
(207) 786-2976
OPEN-AIR/SEASONAL

Augusta Farmers' Market
Wednesday - Water Street
Saturday - Turnpike Mall, Western Avenue
Augusta, ME 04330
Contact: Sharon Carter
(207) 737-2872
OPEN-AIR/SEASONAL

MARYLAND

Baltimore Farmers' Market
Holiday & Saratoga Streets
Baltimore, MD 21202
Contact: Carole Simon
(410) 752-8632
OPEN-AIR/SEASONAL

Southern Maryland Regional Farmers' Market
Route 301 South, state warehouse
Cheltenham, MD 20623
Contact: David Rada
(301) 372-1066 or (in MD) 1-800-533-FARM
SEASONAL

MASSACHUSETTS

Charlton/Mass Pike Farmers' Market
Visitor information service area
Boston, MA 02202
Contact: Anneli Johnson
(617) 727-3018
OPEN-AIR/SEASONAL

Springfield Farmers' Market
Main & E. Court Street, Civic Center
Springfield, MA 01001
(413) 786-9817
Contact: Liz Middleton
OPEN-AIR/SEASONAL

MICHIGAN

Detroit Eastern Market
2934 Russell Street
Detroit, MI 48207
Contact: Jesse Henderson
(313) 833-1560
YEAR-ROUND

Grand Rapids City Farmers' Market II
140 Monroe Center, Suite 300
Grand Rapids, MI 49503
Contact: Debbie Myscka
(616) 774-7124
OPEN-AIR/SEASONAL

MINNESOTA

Minneapolis Farmers' Market
Off Interstate 94, exit 230
Minneapolis, MN 55440
Contact: Larry Cermak
(612) 333-1718
SEASONAL

St. Paul Farmers' Market
290 E. Fifth Street
St. Paul, MN 55101
Contact: Patty Brand
(612) 227-8101
SEASONAL

MISSISSIPPI

Central Farmers' Market
352 Woodrow Wilson
Jackson, MS 39216
Contact: Billy Carter
(601) 354-6573
SEASONAL

Meridian Area Farmers' Market
1800 Main Street
Meridian, MS 39301
Contact: Jim Hollis
(601) 482-9764
SEASONAL

MISSOURI

Jefferson City Farmers' Market
Washington Park
Jefferson City, MO 65101
Contact: Mike Bollinger
(314) 634-6482
OPEN-AIR/SEASONAL

Farmers' Markets — continued

Kansas City Farmers' Market
5th & Main Streets off Interstate 70
Kansas City, MO 64106
Contact: Robin Taylor
(816) 842-1271
YEAR-ROUND

MONTANA

Billings Farmers' Market
4515 Rimrock Road
Billings, MT 59105
Contact: Laura Mitchell
OPEN-AIR/SEASONAL

Helena Farmers' Market
941 Wilder Avenue
Helena, MT 59601
Contact: Betty LaSalle
(406) 442-1355
OPEN-AIR/SEASONAL

NEBRASKA

Lincoln Haymarket Farmers' Market
(2 Locations)
Saturday - Downtown Haymarket District
Wednesday - Foundation Garden, 1417 N Street
Lincoln, NE 68508
Contact: Billene Nemec
(402) 435-7496
OPEN-AIR/SEASONAL

The Omaha Farmers' Market
(2 locations)
Thursday - Old Market parking lot,
11th & Jackson Streets
Saturday - Rockbrook Shopping Center,
108th & Center
Omaha, NE 68131
Contact: Vic Gutman
(402) 345-5401
OPEN-AIR/SEASONAL

NEW HAMPSHIRE

Concord Farmers' Market
North State Street
Concord, NH 03301
Contact: Sherrie Morrill
(603) 753-4849
OPEN-AIR/SEASONAL

NH Farmers' Open Air Market -Manchester
Beech & Valley Streets
Manchester, NH 03104
Contact: Gene Matteuzzi
(603) 432-2978
OPEN-AIR/SEASONAL

NEW JERSEY

Market Square Farmers' Market
275 West Market Street
Newark, NJ 07103
Contact: Authur Coles
(908) 355-5458
OPEN-AIR/SEASONAL

Trenton Farmers' Market
960 Spruce Street
Trenton, NJ 08648
Contact: Jack & Marcia Ball
(609) 695-2998
YEAR-ROUND

NEW MEXICO

Albuquerque Growers' Market
Caravan East parking lot
7605 Central Avenue, N.E.
Albuquerque, NM 87110
Contact: Ed & Pat Shaffer
(505) 265-7250
OPEN-AIR/SEASONAL

Santa Fe Farmers' Market
Sanbusco Market Center
Santa Fe, NM 87505
Contact: Pamela Roy
(505) 983-4098
OPEN-AIR/SEASONAL

NEW YORK

Central New York Regional Farmers' Market
2100 Park Street & Hiawatha Boulevard
Syracuse, NY 13208
Contact: Chris Togias
(315) 422-8647
OPEN-AIR/YEAR-ROUND

East Harlem Community Farmers' Market
98th Street & Lexington Avenue
New York, NY 10029
Contact: Hilary Baum
(718) 884-5716
OPEN-AIR/SEASONAL

Federal Plaza Greenmarket
Broadway & Thomas Streets
New York, NY 10013
Contact: Barry Benepe
(212) 477-3220
OPEN-AIR/YEAR-ROUND

NORTH CAROLINA

North Asheville Tailgate Market
Grace Plaza
Asheville, NC 28801
Contact: Ira Mallard
(704) 683-1812
OPEN-AIR/SEASONAL

Charlotte Regional Farmers' Market
1801 Yorkmont Road, P.O. Box 669184
Charlotte, NC 28266-9184
Contact: Frank Suddreth
(704) 357-1269
YEAR-ROUND

NORTH DAKOTA

Bismarck Farmers' Market
K-mart parking lot
Lincoln, ND 58501
Contact: Richard Kimball
(701) 224-9973
OPEN-AIR/SEASONAL

The Community Farmers' Market
400 4th Street South
Fargo, ND 58103
Contact: Jim Hahn
(701) 347-4933
OPEN-AIR/SEASONAL

OHIO

East Cleveland Farmers' Market
Coit & Woodworth Avenues
Cleveland, OH 44112
Contact: Dick Woodworth
(216) 428-1385
OPEN-AIR/SEASONAL

North Market
29 Spruce Street
Columbus, OH 43215
Contact: Karen Knies
(614) 463-9664
OPEN-AIR/SEASONAL

OKLAHOMA

Farmers Public Market
311 Klein Street
Oklahoma City, OK 73108
Contact: Manager
(405) 232-6506
OPEN-AIR/SEASONAL

Stillwater Main Street Farmers' Market
P.O. Box 1881
Stillwater, OK 74076
Contact: Renee Harris
(405) 624-2921
OPEN-AIR/SEASONAL

OREGON

Lane County Farmers' Market
East 8th & Oak Streets
Eugene, OR 97401
Contact: David Amorose
(503) 342-5856
OPEN-AIR/SEASONAL

Portland Farmers' Market
1200 Northwest Front Avenue
Portland, OR 97215
Contact: Craig Mosbaek
(503) 705-2460
OPEN-AIR/SEASONAL

PENNSYLVANIA

Reading Terminal Market
51 North 12th & Arch Street
Philadelphia, PA 19107
Contact: Gerry Murphy
(215) 922-2317
YEAR-ROUND

State College Farmers' Market
Locust Lane
State College, PA 16801
Contact: Mrs. Scott Case
(814) 422-8735
OPEN-AIR/SEASONAL

RHODE ISLAND

South Kingstown Farmers' Market
Kearney Gym, University of RI, Route 138
Kingston, RI 02881
Contact: Patricia Gardiner
(401) 789-1388
OPEN-AIR/SEASONAL

The Governor Dyer Cooperative Market Inc.
Between Promenade, Valley, Rathbone, and Hemlock Streets
Providence, RI 02908
Contact: Cindy Mello
(401) 273-8800
SEASONAL

SOUTH CAROLINA

Columbia Farmers' Market
P.O. Box 13504
Columbia, SC 29201
Contact: Lee Sowell
(803) 253-4041
YEAR-ROUND

Greenville State Farmers' Market
1354 Rutherford Road
Greenville, SC 29609
Contact: Jack Watson
(803) 244-4023
YEAR-ROUND

SOUTH DAKOTA

Chamber of Commerce Farmers' Market
108 East Missouri Avenue
Pierre, SD 57501
Contact: Gail Brink
(605) 224-7361
OPEN-AIR/SEASONAL

Downtown Farmers' Market, Main Street
415 South 1st Avenue
Sioux Falls, SD 57501
Contact: Beth Knoblock
(605) 338-4009
OPEN-AIR/SEASONAL

TENNESSEE

Knox County Regional Farmers' Market
4700 New Harvest Lane
Knoxville, TN 37918
Contact: Kevin Hosey
(615) 524-3276
YEAR-ROUND

Metro Farmers' Market
618 Jackson Street
Nashville, TN 37219
Contact: Larry Suiter
(615) 259-7903
YEAR-ROUND

TEXAS

San Antonio Farmers' Market
Jackson-Keller Road
San Antonio, TX 78230
Contact: Andy Vidaure
(210) 663-3579
OPEN-AIR/SEASONAL

Farmers' Markets — continued

South Austin Farmers' Market
Pickle Road off South Congress Avenue
Austin, TX 78704
Contact: Anthony Piccola
(512) 285-4758
YEAR-ROUND

UTAH

Downtown Alliance Farmers' Market
Pioneer Park, 300 West & 300 South
Salt Lake City, UT 84111
Contact: Brad Parkin
(801) 359-5118
OPEN-AIR/SEASONAL

Spanish Fork Farmers' Market
City Park, Center & Main Streets
Spanish Fork, UT 84660
Contact: Mary Maslyn
(801) 798-5000
OPEN-AIR/SEASONAL

VERMONT

Capitol City Farmers' Market
State & Elm Street
Montpelier, VT 05601
Contact: Margery Bower
(802) 229-1935
OPEN-AIR/SEASONAL

West River Farmers' Market
Routes 11 & 100
Londonderry, VT 05148
Contact: Ann Hausslein
(802) 824-4486
OPEN-AIR/SEASONAL

VIRGINIA

Charlottesville City Farmers' Market
Carver Recreation Center
Charlottesville, VA 22906
Contact: Bob Crytzer
(804) 971-3271
OPEN-AIR/SEASONAL

Richmond Farmers' Market
17th & Main Streets
Richmond, VA 23232
Contact: Larry Ingram
(804) 780-8597
OPEN-AIR/SEASONAL

WASHINGTON

Pike Place Market
First Avenue & Pike
Seattle, WA 98101
Contact: Steve Evans
(206) 682-7453
OPEN-AIR/SEASONAL

Spokane Marketplace
Riverfront Park
Spokane, WA 99202
Contact: Jackie Rappe
(509) 482-2627
OPEN-AIR/SEASONAL

WEST VIRGINIA

Charleston Farmers' Market
599 Eagan Street
Charleston, WV 25301
Contact: Henry Bender
(304) 558-0185
YEAR-ROUND

Morgantown Farmers' Market
High Street Court House Plaza
Morgantown, WV 26507
Contact: Asel Kennedy
(304) 291-7201
OPEN-AIR/SEASONAL

WISCONSIN

Madison Farmers' Market
Capitol Square
Madison, WI 53714
Contact: Mary Carpenter
(414) 563-5037
OPEN-AIR/SEASONAL

Milwaukee Farmers' Market
4th & Wisconsin Avenue
Milwaukee, WI 53201
Contact: Elizabeth Nicols
(414) 276-6696
OPEN-AIR/SEASONAL

WYOMING

Casper Farmers' Market
2011 Fairgrounds Road
Casper, WY 82604
Contact: Sue Jones
(307) 261-5219
OPEN-AIR/SEASONAL

Cheyenne Farmers' Market
1620 Central Avenue
Cheyenne, WY 82001
Contact: Bill Buckles
(307) 635-9291
OPEN-AIR/SEASONAL

Hotlines, Addresses, Internet

U.S. DEPARTMENT OF AGRICULTURE

TEAM NUTRITION

For more information to get your children's school involved in the promotion of healthy school meals, contact:

USDA's TEAM NUTRITION SCHOOLS
P.O. Box 0812
Rockville, MD 20848-0812
Email:teamnutrition@reeusda.gov

USDA's Food and Nutrition Information Center (FNIC) is located at the USDA's National Agricultural Library in Beltsville, Maryland. USDA program participants may borrow food service reference materials, videos, and training materials free of charge. The public is able to visit the Library and research nutrition education and training materials. On-line bibliographies are offered to assist you in research.

FNIC maintains Gopher and World Wide Web (W W W) sites where users may read, print, or download information. FNIC is linked to other Gopher and WWW sites around the world. The WWW address for FNIC is:

http://www.nal.usda.gov/fnic/

The Gopher address is:

gopher.nal.usda.gov

USDA's Food Safety and Inspection Service offers the

1 (800) 535-4555 Meat and Poultry Hotline

for consumers. Contact the Meat and Poultry Hotline for information on food safety, labeling, and wholesomeness of foods. In Washington, D.C. call 202-720-3333. English and Spanish messages available.

You may write for materials:

USDA Food Safety and Inspection Service
Meat and Poultry Hotline
Room 1165 South Building
Washington, D.C. 20250

U.S. DEPARTMENT OF HEALTH AND HUMAN SERVICES

Food and Drug Administration

FDA/USDA Food Labeling Education Information Center
(301)443-3220

Contact this organization for materials and activities related to food labeling education, or write:

Food and Drug Administration
Office of Public Affairs
5600 Fishers Lane, HFE-88
Rockville, MD 20857

The Food and Drug Administration offers the

1 (800)FDA-4010 Seafood Hotline

for information on seafood buying, handling, and storage for home consumption and labeling. Also provides seafood publications and prerecorded seafood safety messages. In Washington D.C. call (202)205-4314. English and Spanish messages available.

National Health Information Center

1 (800)336-4797
(301)565-4167 (in MD)

Provides a central source of information and referral for health questions from health educators, health professionals, and the public. A service of the Office of Disease Prevention and Health Promotion, U.S. Department of Health and Human Services.

National Health Information Center
P.O. Box 1133
Washington, DC 20013-1133
Fax: (301)984-4256

Hotlines, Addresses, Internet — continued

OTHER ORGANIZATIONS

National Center for Nutrition and Dietetics
1(800)366-1655 Consumer Nutrition Hotline
The American Dietetic Association. Listen to a food and nutrition message, speak to a Registered Dietitian, or for a referral to a Registered Dietitian in your area. English and Spanish messages available.

For more information, write to:
The American Dietetic Association
National Center for Nutrition and Dietetics
216 W. Jackson Blvd.
Chicago, IL 60606-6995

Safe Drinking Water Hotline
1(800)426-4791
U.S. Environmental Protection Agency

Aerobics and Fitness Foundation of America
1(800)233-4886
Answers questions from the public regarding safe and effective exercise programs and practices.

American Institute for Cancer Research
1(800)843-8114
Provides free educational publications about diet, nutrition, and cancer prevention, as well as a Nutrition Hotline staffed by Registered Dietitians.

Cancer Information Service
1(800)4-CANCER
Provides information about cancer and related resources to the public. Distributes free publications from the National Cancer Institute.

Combined Health Information Database (CHID)
1(800)955-0906
(BRS Online, to subscribe to CHID)
Database contains many diverse health education resources. It may be accessed at many university, medical, and public libraries.

Consumer Information Center
General Services Administration
P.O. Box 100
Pueblo, CO 81009
(719)948-4000
Distributes Federal agency publications. Publishes quarterly catalog of available materials.

Centers for Disease Control and Prevention
National Center for Chronic Disease Prevention and Health Promotion (NCCDPHP)
Technical Information Service Branch
4770 Buford Highway, MS K13
Atlanta, FA 30341-3724
(404)488-5080

Provides information and referrals to the public and to professionals. Visit the NCCDPHP Information Center and use the collection by appointment.

National Dairy Council
1(800)426-8271
Develops and provides educational materials on nutrition.

Women's Sports Foundation
1(800)227-3988
Provides information on women's sports, physical fitness, and sports medicine.

National Heart, Lung, and Blood Institute
Information Center (NHLBI)
P.O. Box 30105
Bethesda, MD 2024-0105
(301)251-1222
(301)251-1223 (Fax)
Materials on cardiovascular health are available to consumers and professionals.

National Center for Education in Maternal and Child Health
2000 North 15th Street
Suite 701
Arlington, VA 22201-7802
(703)524-7802
(703)524-9335 (Fax)
Responds to information requests form consumers and professionals, provides technical assistance, and develops educational and reference materials.

National Maternal and Child Health Clearinghouse
8201 Greensboro Drive
Suite 600
McLean, VA 22102
(703)821-8955, ext 254 or 265
(703)821-2098 (Fax)
Centralized source of materials and information in the areas of human genetics and maternal and child health. Distributes publications and provides referrals.

National Restaurant Association The Educational Foundation
Industry Council on Food Safety
1(800)-COOK-SMART
1(800-266-5762
Provides information on safe food preparation and handling.

President's Council on Physical Fitness and Sports
701 Pennsylvania Avenue NW.
Suite 250
Washington, DC 20004
(202)272-3430
(202)504-2064 (Fax)
Materials on exercise and physical fitness for all ages are available.

U.S. Consumer Product Safety Commission Hotline
Washington, DC
1(800)638-2772
1(800)638-8270 (TT)
(301)504-0580
(301)504-0399 (Fax)
Maintains the National Injury Information Clearinghouse. Maintains free hotline to provide information about recalls and to receive reports on unsafe products and product-related injuries.

USDA's Team Nutrition Supporters

To date, over 300 organizations, including nutrition, health, education, entertainment, and food industry groups support Team Nutrition's Mission and Principles.

THESE ORGANIZATIONS SUPPORT THE MISSION AND PRINCIPLES OF TEAM NUTRITION

ADVOCAP, Inc.
Agricultural Women's Leadership Network
Agenda for Children
Albany Park Community Center
Alivio Medical Center
American Academy of Pediatrics
American Alliance for Health, PE. Rec. & Dance
American Association of Family & Consumer Sciences
American Bakers Association
American Cancer Society
American College of Physicians
American College of Preventive Medicine
American Culinary Federation
American Dietetic Association
American Farm Bureau Federation
American Federation of School Administrators
American Federation of Teachers
American Fine Foods
American Health Foundation
American Heart Association
American Heart Association, MD Affiliate
American Institute for Cancer Research
American Institute of Wine & Food
American Meat Institute
American Medical Association
American Medical Student Association
American National CattleWomen, Inc.
American Nurses Association
American Oat Association
American Psychological Association
American Public Health Association
American School Food Service Association
Archer Daniels Midland Company
Archway Cookies
Arkansas Poultry Federation/Egg Council
Association for Child Development
Associated Churches Food Bank System
Association for Children of New Jersey
Association for the Advancement of Health Education
Association of Maternal & Child Health Programs
Association of State and Territorial Public Health Nutrition Directors, ASTPHND
Auglaize Mercer CAC
Aurora Project., Inc.
Beef Products
Bennington-Rutland Opportunity Council (BROC)
Better Baked Pizza, Inc.
Big Brothers/Big Sisters of America
Blue Diamond Growers
Boy Scouts of America
Bread for the World
Brooks Foods
Bumble Bee Seafoods, Inc.
California Apricot Advisory Board
California Beef Council
California Department of Education
California Food Policy Advocates
California Fresh Carrot Advisory Board
California Prune Board
California Tomato Growers Association
Campaign for Food Literacy
Camp Fire, First Texas Council
Cancer Research Foundation of America
Careers Through Culinary Arts Program
Center for Environmental Education
Center for Science in the Public Interest
Center on Hunger, Poverty & Nutrition Policy/Tufts University School of Nutrition
Cherry Marketing Institute
Children's Action Alliance
Children's Action Network
Children's Defense Fund
Children's Foundation
Citizens for Missouri's Children
Citizens for Public Action on Blood Pressure & Cholesterol
City of Columbus, Health Department
City of Rockford (IL) Head Start Program
Colorado PTA
Community & Economic Development Association (CEDA) WIC Program
Community Kitchen of Monroe County, Inc.
Community Resource Center (OH)
Comstock Michigan Fruits
ConAgra, Inc.
Congressional Hunger Center
Consumer Federation of America
Cooperative State Research, Education & Extension Service, USDA
Corning Consumer Products Company
Council of Agricultural Science & Technology
Council of the Great City Schools
Culinary Institute of America
Curtice Burns Foods
Diet Workshop
DINE Systems
Dole Food Company, Inc.
Draper King Cole, Inc.
Eastern Shore Seafoods Products
Eastside Community Ministry
Education Council
EHOVE Career Center (OH)

Family Nutrition Program/Purdue University Cooperative Extension Service
Fimast Supermarkets
Fine CAP Inc.
Finger Lakes Packaging
Florida Department of Citrus
FOCUS:HOPE
Food Bank of Oakland Country (MI)
Food Chain
Food Marketing Institute
Food Research & Action Center
Foodservice Systems Management
Food to Grow Coalition
Furman Foods, Inc.
Gehl's Guernsey Farms, Inc.
General Mills, Inc.
Georgia Department of Agriculture
Giant Food Inc.
Gilroy Canning Company, Inc.
Girl Scouts of the USA
Girl Scouts - Mile Hi Council
Gleaners Foodbank of Indiana, Inc.
Green Thumb, Inc.
Health Matters!
HJ Heinz Company
Hormel Foods Corporation
House of Mercy Daycare
Howard Foods, Inc.
Hudson Specialty Foods
Hunger Action Coalition
Husman Snack Foods
Illinois Community Action Association
Illinois Department of Agriculture
Illinois State Horticultural Society
Indiana Agricutural Leadership Institute
Indiana State Univ. — Department of Family & Consumer Sciences
International Apple Institute
International Food Information Council
International Food Service Distributors Association
J.R. Simplot Co.
James Beard Foundation/Dando & Company
Jewish Healthcare Foundation of Pittsburgh
Johnson & Wales University
Kankakee County WIC Program
Kelly Foods, Inc.
Kent State University, School of Family and Consumer Studies
KIDSNET
Lakeside Foods, Inc.
Land O'Lakes Custom Products Division
LDS Church Welfare Services
Life Lab Science Program
MAGNAtracker Company
Maudester Farmer
Marriott Management Services
Maternal — Child Health Center (IN)
Marvel Entertainment Group
Mello Smello
Memorial Medical Center (IL)
Michigan Apple Committee
Michigan Asparagus Advisory Board
Michigan Plum Advisory Board
Michigan Red Tart Cherry Information Committee
Middlesex Co. — Vocational Technical High School
Mid-Ohio Foodbank
Minnesota Cultivated Wild Rice Council
Minnesota Food Education & Resource Center
Minnesota Food Share
Mothers & Others
Muir Glen Organic Tomato Products
Nalley's Fine Foods
National 4-H Council
National Alliance of Vietnamese-American Service Agencies
National American Wholesale Grocers Association
National Association for Sport & Physical Education
National Association of Elementary School Principals
National Association of Psychiatric
Treatment Centers for Children
National Association of School Nurses
National Association of School Psychologists
National Association of State NET Coordinators
National Association of WIC Directors
National Black Child Development Institute
National Black Nurses Association
National Black Women's Health Project
National Broiler Council
National Cancer Institute
National Cattlemen's Beef Association
National Consumers League
National Council of LaRaza
National Dairy Council
Dairy Council of Central States
Dairy Council Mid East
Washington State Dairy Council
National Dental Association
National Dry Bean Council
National Education Association
National Extension Association of Family and Consumer Sciences
National Farmers Organization
National Farmers Union
National Fisheries Institute
National Fitness Leaders Association
National Food Service Management Institute
National Future Farmers of America
National Gardening Association
National Grange
National Heart Savers Association

National Medical Association
National Osteoporosis Foundation
National Pasta Association
National Pork Producers Council
National PTA
National Puerto Rican Coalition
National Restaurant Association
National Rural Electric Cooperative Association
National School Health Education Coalition
National Turkey Federation
National Urban League
New England Dairy Food Council
New Hampshire Fruit Growers Association
North Atlantic Sardine Council
North Carolina Sweet Potato Commission
Northeast McIntosh Growers Association
Northwestern University Settlement
Nutrition Council of Greater Cincinnati
Nutrition Education Learning Lab
Ocean Spray Cranberries, Inc.
Ohio Hunger Task Force
Orange County WIC/Child Health Project
Ore-Ida Foods, Inc.
Organization of Chinese Americans
Our Daily Bread
Pennsylvania Coalition on Food & Nutrition
Perdue Farms, Inc.
Physical Rehabilitation & Health Center
Pomptonian School Food Service
Post Bulletin (MN)
Potato Board
President's Council on Physical Fitness & Sports
Procter & Gamble Company
Produce for Better Health Foundation (5-A-Day)
Produce Business
Produce Marketing Association
Produce Productions, Inc.
Project NOW Community Action Agency
Public Voice for Food & Health Policy
Pumpkin Circle
Quaker Oats Company
Randall Foods Products, Inc.
RC Fine Foods
Sabatasso Foods, Inc.
Salvation Army of Greater Cleveland (OH)
Scholastic, Inc.
Second Harvest National Foodbank Network
Second Harvest - St. Paul
Second Harvest - Tri-State Food Bank, Inc.
Seward Dairy, Inc.
Shape Up America
Share Our Strength
Simpson Housing Services
Snyder of Berlin
Society for Nutrition Education
Society of State Directors of Health, Physical Education and Recreation
Soup Kitchen of Minnesota
Southeast Alaska Health Consortium
Southern Frozen Foods
Soy Protein Council
Squab Producers of California
St. Francis Soup Kitchen (OH)
Sugar Association
Sunkist Growers, Inc.
Sunshine Biscuits
Texas Citrus & Vegetable Association
Texas Produce Association
Tim's Cascade Chips
Tony's Food Service Division
Tone's
Townsend Culinary, Inc.
Tree Top, Inc.
United Soybean Council
United States Department of Education
United States Department of Health & Human Services
United Way of Monroe County (IN)
University Extension, University of Missouri
University Extension, Schuyler County
University of Cincinnati Nutrition Program & Nutrition Learning Center
University of Hawaii Cooperative Extension Service
Urban Coalition
Urban Family Institute
Urban Mission
USA Dry Pea & Lentil Council
USA Rice Federation
USA TODAY
Van Camp Seafood Company, Inc.
Vegetarian Resource Group
Virginia Apple Growers Association
Voices for Children in Nebraska
Walnut Hills/Over The Rhine Kitchen
Walt Disney Company
Warren County (OH) Head Start
Wawona Frozen Foods
West Virginia Association of Family & Consumer Science
West Virginia WIC Program
Wheat Foods Council
Wisconsin Nutrition Project
Wisconsin Rural Development Center, Inc.
World Hunger Year (Kids Can Make A Difference)
Wyoming Extension
Zartic, Inc.

Team Nutrition is a program of the United States Department of Agriculture. USDA does not endorse any products, services, or organizations.

Team Nutrition Supporters' Resources for Family Use

The following organizations have materials available to share with you and your family on nutrition, recipes, food handling and safety in the kitchen, etc. Feel free to contact or write to them for more information:

Please note: *Unless otherwise noted, there may be a small charge for materials from some organizations. Team Nutrition is a program of the United States Department of Agriculture. USDA does not endorse any products, services, or organizations.*

ADVOCAP, Inc. Agenda for Children
PO Box 1108
Fond du Lac, WI 54936
phone: 414-922-7760
Nutrition education activities, publications, information on Hunger Prevention Coalition, Head Start Program.

Agenda For Children
Child Care Resources/ Positive Steps Training Team
Training Program Coordinator
PO Box 51837
New Orleans, LA 70151
phone: 504-586-8509
workshops

Agricultural Women's Leadership Network
President
Drawer 88
Kilgore, NE 69216-0088
phone:402-966-2741
recipes/cooking information; nutrition education activities

American Academy of Pediatrics
Department C-PRG
PO Box 927
Elk Grove Village, IL 60009-0927
publication: Parent Resource Guide listing nutrition brochures available

American Bakers Association
1350 I St., NW
Suite 1290
Washington, DC 20005-3305
phone: 202-789-0300
publications, other-information regarding American Bakers Association National Nutrition Education Program for Bread & Rolls

American Culinary Federation
10 San Bartola Drive
St. Augustine, FL 32086
phone: 800-624-9458
recipes/publications/books

American Fine Foods, Inc.
Research Coordinator
PO Box 460
Payette, ID 83661
phone: 208-642-6340
Nutrition Facts interpretation

American Health Foundation
320 E. 43rd St.
New York, NY 10017
nutrition education activities

American Heart Association
7272 Greenville Avenue
Dallas, TX 75231-4596
phone:1-800-AHA-USA1
email:http://www.amhrt.org
for information about heart-health, or to learn how the new AHA Schoolsite Program - HeartPower! can help your children be heart-healthy for a lifetime

American Heart Association, MD Affiliate
415 N. Charles St.
Baltimore, MD 21203
phone: 410-685-7074
recipes, nutrition education activities, publications

American Institute for Cancer Research
1759 R St., NW
Washington, DC 20009
Nutrition Hotline: 1-800-743-8114
recipes, nutrition education activities, publications, (nutrition and cancer prevention) and health aids dealing with nutrition and diet

American Institute of Wine & Food
1550 Bryant St.
San Francisco, CA 94103
phone: 415-255-3000
publications: AIWF Standards Document, AIWF Newsletter

Resources for Family Use — continued

American National CattleWomen, Inc.
PO Box 3881
Englewood, CO 80016
phone: 303-694-0313
National Beef Cook-Off Information and National Beef Ambassador Contest Information

American Oat Association
415 Shelard Parkway
Suite 101
Minneapolis, MN 55426
phone: 612-542-9817
recipes/cooking information; publications ("OatFoods: A Smart Choice" brochure)

American Psychological Association
750 First Street, NE
Washington, DC 20002
publications

Archway Cookies, Inc.
5451 West Dickman Road
PO Box 762
Battle Creek, MI 49016-0762
phone: 616-962-6205
recipes/cooking information; nutrition education activities

Association for Advancement of Health Education
(an organization with American Alliance for Health, PE, Recreation & Dance)
Program Administrator
1900 Association Drive
Reston, VA 22091
nutrition education activities; publications (eating disorders, computerized nutrition analyses)

Association for Children of New Jersey
35 Halsey Street
Newark, NJ 07102
phone: 201-643-3876
publication "Families in Focus"

Association of Maternal & Child Health Programs
(MA Dept. of Public Health)
Bureau of Family & Community Health
250 Washington Street, 5th floor
Boston, MA 02108-4619
phone: 1-800-645-8333 (for information on food resources)
phone: 1-800-WIC-1007 (for information on WIC Program)
phone: 1-800-95BONES (for information on osteoporosis)
nutrition education activities, publications (5-A-Day materials, osteoporosis pamphlets, Food Stamp information) other (referrals to WIC, Food Stamps, other food resources)

Association of State & Territorial Public Health Nutrition Directors (ASTPHND)
415 Second St., NE
Suite 200
Washington, DC 20002
phone: 202-546-2630
email:prob101w@wonder.em.cdc.gov
referrals to state & local nutrition programs

Aurora Project, Inc.
1035 North Superior St.
Toledo, OH 43604
phone: 419-244-3200
recipes, nutrition information, outreach to homeless women & children

Beef Products, Inc.
891 Two Rivers Drive
Dakota Dunes, SD 57049
recipes/cooking information, nutrition education activities

Better Baked Pizza, Inc.
12340 Gay Road
North East, PA 16428
phone: 814-725-8498
nutrition education activities

California Apricot Advisory Board
Assistant Manager
1280 Boulevard Way
Suite 107
Walnut Creek, CA 94595-1154
phone: 510-937-3660
recipes/cooking information, nutrition education activities

California Beef Council
Materials Coordinator
(state of CA only)
551 Foster City Blvd.
Suite A
Foster City, CA 94404
phone: 415-571-7100
email: calbeef@ix.netcom.com
recipes/cooking information, nutrition education activities

California Department of Education, Child Nutrition & Food Distribution Division
560 J Street
Suite 270
Sacramento, CA 95814
phone: 1-800-952-5609
email:Mbriggs@cde.ca.gov
recipes/cooking information, nutrition education activities, publications

California Fresh Carrot Advisory Board
531 D North Alta Avenue
Dinuba, CA 93618
phone:209-591-4725
recipes/cooking information

California Prune Board
Suite 101
5990 Stoneridge Dr.
Pleasanton, CA 94588
phone: 510-734-0150
recipes/cooking information

California Tomato Growers Association
2529 W. March Lane
Suite 204
PO Box 7398
Stockton, CA 95267-0398
email: growers@tomato.com
recipes/cooking information, nutrition education activities, publication - The California Tomato Grower magazine ($30.00 per year subscription in US)

The Campaign for Food Literacy
3721 Midvale Ave.
Philadelphia, PA 19129
phone: 215-951-0330
publications

Cancer Research Foundation of America
Director of Programs
200 Daingerfield Rd.
Alexandria, VA 22314
phone:1-800-227-CRFA
recipes/cooking information, nutrition education activities, publications (Cancer Research Foundation Guide to Healthy Eating), CD-ROM game Dr. Health'snstein's Body Fun

Careers Through Culinary Arts Program, Inc.
Program Director
155 W. 68th St.
New York, NY 10023
phone: 212-873-2434
email:ccap inc@aol.com
teaches high-school students entry level skills for chefs; offers scholarships, hospitality

Center for Environmental Education
Librarian
400 Columbus Avenue
Valhalla, NY 10595
phone: 914-747-8200
email:cee@earthspint.org
nutrition education activities

Cherry Marketing Institute
2220 University Park Drive
Okemos, MI 48864
phone: 517-347-0010
recipes/cooking information, nutrition education activities

The Children's Foundation
725 15th St., NW
Suite 505
Washington, DC 20005-2109
email:CF washdc@aol.com
publications, Child Nutrition Information: Birth - 6 years

Community Kitchen of Monroe County, Inc.
917 S. Rogers
Bloomington, IL 47403
phone: 812-332-0999

The Congressional Hunger Center
525 A Street, NE
Suite 308
Washington, DC 20002
phone: 202-547-7022
email:HN3228@handsnet.org
nutrition education activities, hunger related activities

Resources for Family Use — continued

DINE Systems
586 North French Road
Amherst, NY 14228
phone: 716-688-2400
email: DINESystem@aol.com
nutrition education activities and software; nutrition software

Eastern Shore Seafood
PO Box 38
Mappsville, VA 23407
phone: 1-800-446-8550
recipes/cooking information

Eastside Community Ministry
40 N. 6th Street
Zangsville, OH 43701
recipes, nutrition education activities, publications

Family Nutrition Program
Purdue University Cooperative Extension Service
1260 MTHW
Purdue University
West Lafayette, IN 47907
phone: 317-496-2488
email: claryj@sage.cc.purdue.edu
recipes, nutrition education activities, publications, other (individual or group lessons, food demonstrations, videos)

Florida Department of Citrus
Foodservice Business Unit
PO Box 148
Lakeland, FL 33802
phone: 941-499-2457
recipes/cooking information

Food Marketing Institute
800 Connecticut Ave., NW
Washington, DC 20006
email:fmi@fmi.org
recipes/cooking information, nutrition education activities, publications (charges will apply)

Georgia Dept. of Agriculture
328 Agriculture Bldg.
Atlanta, GA 30334
phone: 404-656-3678
in GA only: 1-800-282-5852 x3678
recipes, publications (Commodity fact sheets, 5-A-Day brochure - Fruits & Vegetables)

Gleaners Food Bank of Indiana, Inc.
1102 E. 16th Street
Indianapolis, IN 46202-1944
phone: 1-800-944-9166
publications, other (newsletter from "The Indiana Food & Nutrition Network")

Green Thumb, Inc.
2000 N. 14th St.
Suite 800
Arlington, VA 22201
recipes/cooking information

Hormel Foods Corporation
Manager, Consumer Response
1 Hormel Place
Austin, MN 55912
phone: 1-800-523-4635
recipes/cooking information; nutrition information

Hunger Action Coalition
220 Bagley
Suite 326
Detroit, MI 48226
email: Hno144@handsnet.org
nutrition education activities, publications (Bring on Breakfast), resource and referral information, technical assistance in helping to start food pantries, community organizing, resource development, advocacy for nutrition programs

International Apple Institute
6707 Old Dominion Dr.
Suite 320
McLean, VA 22101
recipes, nutrition education, publications. (Please include a self-addressed stamped envelope with request)

Michigan Apple Committee
13105 Schavey Road
Suite 5
Dewitt, MI 48820
phone: 1-800-456-2753

Michigan Asparagus Advisory Board
2133 University Park Drive
Suite 700
Okemos, MI 48864-5909
recipes/cooking information, nutrition education activities

Michigan Plum Advisory Board
2133 University Park Drive
Suite 700
Okemos, MI 48864-5909
recipes/cooking information, nutrition education activities

Minnesota Cultivated Wild Rice Council
1306 County Road F
Suite 109
St. Paul, MN 55112
phone: 1-800-235-8906
recipes/cooking information; information regarding wild rice as a farm crop

Minnesota Food Share
122 W. Franklin Avenue
Suite 218
Minneapolis, MN 55404
phone: 612-870-3660
publications

Mothers & Others for a Liveable Planet
40 W. 20th St.
New York, NY 10011
email: mothers@rgc.apc.org
recipes, nutrition education activities, publications

Muir Glen Organic Tomato Products
424 North 7th St.
Sacramento, CA 95814
phone: 1-800-832-6345
recipes/cooking information; nutrition information

National 4-H Council
7100 Connecticut Ave.
Chevy Chase, MD 20815
email: sans%smtpgatedfourthcouncil.edu
publications; name & address of the 4-H office in your community

National Association of Psychiatric Treatment Centers for Children
2000 L St., NW
Washington, DC 20036
phone: 202-955-3828
publications

National Association for Sport & Physical Education
1900 Association Drive
Reston, VA 22091
email: naspe@aahperd.org
physical activity information

National Association of WIC Directors
1627 Connecticut Ave., NW
Suite 101
Washington, DC 20009
phone: 202-232-5492
contact information for your state or local WIC agency

National Black Child Development Institute
1023 15th St., NW
Washington, DC 20005
phone: 1- 800-556-2234
nutrition education activities (Nutrition Public Education Campaign), publications (Child Health Talk)

National Dairy Council
10255 W. Higgins Road
Suite 900
Rosemont, IL 60018
phone: 1-800-426-8271
recipes/cooking information, nutrition education activities, publications

National Dairy Council -
Dairy Council Mid East
9380 McKnight Road
Suite 106A
Pittsburgh, PA 15237-5953
phone: 412-367-9120
nutrition education activities

Dairy Council - Washington State
4201 198th Street, SW
Suite 102
Lynnwood, WA 98036
fax: 1-800-470-1222
email:eatwell@ix.netcom.com
publications (materials catalog), educators/health professional resources

Resources for Family Use — continued

National Farmers Union
11900 E. Cornell Avenue
Aurora, CO 80014-3194
phone: 1-800-347-1961
publications (information agriculture/nutrition policy)

National Fisheries Institute
1901 North Fort Myer Dr.
Suite 700
Arlington, VA 22209
email: fishery@ix.netcom.com
recipes, publications

National Fitness Leaders Association
7929 W. Park Dr.
Suite 200
McLean, VA 22102
phone: 703-790-9605
email: nflamj@aol.com
Youth Fitness and Family Fitness brochures

National Food Service Management Institute
University of Mississippi
PO Box 188
Oxford, MS 38677
phone: 1-800-321-3054
email: nfsmi@sunset.backbone.olemiss.edu
recipes/cooking information, nutrition education activities

National Osteoporosis Foundation
1150 17th Street, NW
Suite 500
Washington, DC 20036
phone: 202-223-2226

National Pasta Association
2101 Wilson Blvd.
Suite 920
Arlington, VA 22201
phone: 703-468-5506
email: 103006.16@compuserve.com
http://www.ilovepasta.org
recipes/cooking information, nutrition education activities

National PTA
330 North Wabash Avenue
Suite 2100
Chicago, IL 60611-3690
phone: 312-670-6782
publications, "Our Children" magazine
Contact your state or local PTA.

National Turkey Federation
1225 New York Ave., NW
Washington, DC 20005
phone: 202-898-0100
recipes/cooking information

North Carolina Sweet Potato Commission
1327 Brightleaf Blvd.
Suite H
Smithfield, NC 27577
phone: 919-989-7327
recipes/cooking information

Nutrition Council
2400 Reading Road
Suite 201-B
Cincinnati, OH 45202
phone: 513-621-3262
email: nutri@eos.net
recipes, nutrition education activities, publications (fact sheets, newsletters)

Ocean Spray Cranberries, Inc.
One Ocean Spray Drive
Lakeville, MA 02349
phone: 508-946-7476
email: mrood@oceanspray.com
recipes/cooking information, nutrition education activities, publications

Orange County WIC
Child Health Project
204 E. Main St.
Paoli, IN 47454
phone: 812-723-4131
recipes, nutrition education activities

Ore-Ida Foods
220 W. ParkCenter Blvd.
Boise, ID 83706
phone: 208-383-6286
recipes/cooking information

Perdue Farms
PO Box 708TN
Spring House, PA 19477
Perdue Nutrition Guides, nutrition education curriculum for grade K-3, reference books, and Delicious, Yet Nutritious Recipes

President's Council on Physical Fitness & Sports
701 Pennsylvania Ave., NW
Suite 250
Washington, DC 20004
phone: 202-272-3425
email: cspain@osophs.ssw.dhhs.gov
physical activity and fitness information

Produce Productions, Inc.
PO Box 3556
Cherry Hill, NJ 08034
"The Produce Tip of the Day" - with Greengrocer Johnny Lerro television show - nationally syndicated

Public Voice for Food & Health Policy
1101 14th Street, NW
Suite 710
Washington, DC 20005
phone: 202-371-1840
email: pvoice@tx.netcom.com
publications: recipes, booklets, and reports.

RC Fine Foods
Chef Dimitrious
PO Box 236
Belle Mead, NJ 08502-0236
phone:908-359-5500
recipes, nutrition education activities (lecturer demonstration), American Culinary Federation resource

Second Harvest -St. Paul
1140 Gervais Ave.
St. Paul, MN 55109
email: mn1889igc.org
Foodbank recipes, nutrition education activities

Second Harvest - Tri-State Foodbank, Inc.
801 E. Michigan St.
Evansville, IN 47711-5631
phone: 812-425-0775
recipes, staff consultation, supplemental food

Southeast Alaska Regional Health Consortium
222 Tongass Drive
Sitka, AK 99835
phone: 907-966-8736
recipes/cooking information, nutrition education activities

Soy Protein Council
1255 23rd Street, NW
Suite 850
Washington, DC 20037
phone: 202-467-6610
fact sheet - 50 page booklet on soy in foods

The Sugar Association
1101 15th St., NW
Washington, DC 20005
phone: 202-785-1122
email: sugar@sugar.org
recipes/cooking information, nutrition education activities, Label Power (game teaches food label, ages 9-11), publications (Winning Box Lunches, Pleasing Picky Eaters)

Tony's Food Service
Division Manager
115 W. College Drive
Marshall, MN 56258
phone: 1-800-328-7556
nutrition education activities

United Soybean Board
c/o R. Kehoe
N. Chapman Associates, Inc.
1723 U St., NW
Washington, DC 20009
email: kehoer@aol.com
recipes/cooking information

University of Cincinnati Nutrition Program & Nutrition Learning Center
435 Teachers College
University of Cincinnati
Cincinnati, OH 45221-0022
phone: 513-556-3848
recipes, nutrition education activities, publications

Resources for Family Use — continued

University of Hawaii
Cooperative Extension Service
1920 Edmondson Rd.
Honolulu, HI 96822
phone: 808-956-3842 ext. 6457
email: trish@hawaii.edu
publications, answers to specific nutrition questions

The Urban Mission
Education Coordinator
301 North Fifth St.
Steubenville, OH 43952-2015
phone: 614-282-8010
recipes, nutrition education activities, publications

USA Dry Pea & Lentil Council
5071 Highway 8 West
Moscow, ID 83843
phone: 208-882-3023
recipes/cooking information, nutrition education activities

USA Rice Federation
PO Box 74021
Houston, TX 77274
email: maryjo@tx.usarice.com
fact sheets, brochures (ex. Walking for Fitness), recipes, nutrition education activities

Vegetarian Resource Group
PO Box 1463
Baltimore, MD 21203
phone: 410-366-8343
email: TheVRG@aol.com
recipes/cooking information, many different brochures for all age groups

Virginia Apple Growers Association
1100 Bank Street
Suite 1008
Richmond, VA 23219
phone: 804-371-6104
recipes

Wawona Frozen Foods
100 W. Alluvial
Clovis, CA 93611
1-800-669-2966
email: W-WAWONA
recipes/cooking information

Wheat Foods Council
Office Manager
5500 S. Quebec St.
Englewood, CO 80111
phone: 303-694-5828
Nutrition Education (at cost) - call for an order form

Wisconsin Rural Development Center, Inc.
125 Brookwood Drive
Mount Herob, WI 53572
phone: 608-437-5971
recipes/cookbook (community supported agriculture chapter)

World Hunger Year/USDA's National Clearinghouse
Clearinghouse Manager
505 8th Avenue
New York, NY 10018-6582
phone: 1-800-453-2648
database on nutrition/hunger related organization; also serves as USDA's national clearinghouse

Careful in the Kitchen

Keep hot foods HOT! (Keep food at 140°F or above)

Keep cold foods COLD! (Refrigerate or chill food at 40°F or below)

Keep frozen foods in a freezer at 0°F or lower.

Cook meats such as beef, pork, poultry, and fish to proper internal temperatures. Use a meat thermometer when roasting meats. Juices should run clear and meat should not be pink. Fish should flake easily when tested with a fork.

Do not partially cook food one day and complete cooking the next day.

Set conventional oven temperature to a minimum of 325°F.

Prepare sandwiches and salads with a minimum amount of handling.

Promptly refrigerate or freeze leftovers. Divide large quantities into smaller containers or use shallow pans, for quick cooling.

Reheat leftovers to at least 165°F.

Thaw poultry and meat in a refrigerator. Use thawed roasts, steaks, and chops within three to five days. Use thawed ground beef and poultry within 1 to 2 days. Use hot dogs, ham slices, and luncheon meats within 3 to 5 days. Refreeze only if ice crystals are still present.

Remember USDA's Two-Hour Rule: **Never leave food out at room temperature for more than 2 hours.**

Foods can be placed in the refrigerator hot. Do not leave at room temperature "to cool"; this practice invites bacteria and is unsafe.

Marinate food in the refrigerator, not at room temperature.

Remember that you cannot determine food safety by sight, taste, odor, or smell. If there is any doubt, throw the food away.

Follow instructions exactly on how to use and clean kitchen equipment.

Keep a fire extinguisher and first-aid kit handy.

How Long Should I Keep Food?

Cold Storage Chart

PRODUCT	REFRIGERATOR (40°F)	FREEZER (0°F)
Eggs		
Fresh, in shell	3 weeks	Don't freeze
Raw yolks, whites	2-4 days	1 year
Hardcooked	1 week	Don't freeze well
Liquid pasteurized eggs, or egg substitutes		
opened	3 days	Don't freeze
unopened	10 days	1 year
Meat, Fresh		
Beef	3-5 days	6-12 months
Pork	3-5 days	4-6 months
Veal	3-5 days	4-6 months
Hamburger, Ground and Stew Meats		
Hamburger and Stew meat	1-2 days	3-4 months
Ground turkey, veal, pork, lamb, and mixture of them	1-2 days	3-4 months
Meat Leftovers, Cooked		
Cooked meat and meat dishes	3-4 days	2-3 months
Gravy and meat broth	1-2 days	2-3 months

Adapted from *A Quick Consumer Guide to Safe Food Handling,* Home and Garden Bulletin, No. 248.

PRODUCT	REFRIGERATOR (40°F)	FREEZER (0°F)
Poultry, Fresh		
Chicken or turkey, whole	1-2 days	1 year
Chicken or turkey pieces	1-2 days	9 months
Poultry Leftovers, Cooked		
Cooked poultry dishes	3-4 days	4-6 months
Pieces, plain	3-4 days	4 months
Pieces covered with broth, gravy	1-2 days	6 months
Chicken nuggets, patties	1-2 days	1-3 months
Fried chicken	3-4 days	4 months
Hotdogs & Lunch Meats		
Hotdogs, opened package	1 week	
unopened package	2 weeks	In freezer wrap
Lunch meats, opened	3-5 days	1-2 months
unopened package	2 weeks	
Soups and Stews		
Vegetable or meat-added	3-4 days	2-3 months
Mayonnaise, commercial		
Refrigerate after opening	2 months	Don't freeze
Prepared Salads		
Tuna, ham, macaroni, egg or chicken	3-5 days	Don't freeze well

Books, Pamphlets, Brochures

Nutrition and Your Health: Dietary Guidelines for Americans, Fourth Edition, 1995, U.S. Department of Agriculture and U.S. Department of Health and Human Services.
For sale by the U.S. Government Printing Office, Washington, DC.

Making Healthy Food Choices, USDA, Human Nutrition Information Service, Home & Garden bulletin, No. 250, February 1993, Spanish version, December 1994).
For sale by the U.S. Government Printing Office, Washington, DC.

Preparing Foods and Planning Menus Using the Dietary Guidelines, USDA, Human Nutrition Information Service, Home and Garden Bulletin No. 232-8.
For sale by the U.S. Government Printing Office, Washington, DC.

Food Facts for Older Adults, Information on How to Use the Dietary Guidelines, USDA, Human Nutrition Information Service, Home and Garden Bulletin, No. 251, 1993.
For sale by the U.S. Government Printing Office, Washington, DC.

A Quick Consumer Guide to Safe Food Handling, USDA, Food Safety and Inspection Service, Home and Garden Bulletin, No. 248, 1990.
Contact the USDA Meat & Poultry Hotline, at 1-800-535-4555.

Preventing Foodborne Illness, A Guide to Safe Food Handling, USDA, Food Safety and Inspection Service, Home and Garden Bulletin No. 247, September 1990.
Contact the USDA Meat & Poultry Hotline, at 1-800-535-4555.

The Food Guide Pyramid, USDA/Human Nutrition Information Service, Home and Garden Bulletin No. 252, October 1996.
Available from the Consumer Information Center, Pueblo, CO.

Check It Out, The Food Label, The Pyramid, and You, U.S. Department of Agriculture, Home and Garden Bulletin No. 266, 1994
For sale by the U.S. Government Printing Office, Washington, DC.

Down Home Healthy Cookin' Recipes and Healthy Cooking Tips, March 1995.
Available from the U.S. Department of Health and Human Services, National Institutes of Health National Cancer Institute, NIH publication No. 95-3408SV.

A Tool Kit for Healthy School Meals: Recipes and Training Materials, USDA's New School Lunch and Breakfast Recipes, USDA, Food and Consumer Service, 1995. *Available at school districts and schools who participate in the National School Lunch Program. For sale by the U.S. Government Printing Office, Washington, DC.*

How to Get Involved with Team Nutrition

Want to join Team Nutrition? The first step is to ask your children's principal if the school is, or has plans to become, a Team Nutrition School. If they are not yet a Team Nutrition School, suggest they contact the child nutrition director at your state department of education who can help them get on board. All parents can be a part of Team Nutrition to improve school lunches. You can also be part of your school's nutrition education activities. Try this:

- *Do Lunch With the Kids.* Eat breakfast or lunch at school with your kids. See what the meals are like. Notice the atmosphere. If you want to improve what you see, do something.
- *Talk Out of School.* Make your opinions heard. Talk to other parents. Work with your PTA and school board to support healthy school meals.
- *Discuss Your Principles.* Go to the principal. Discuss the importance of good nutrition and physical activity. Suggest programs. Ask for cooperation. Follow through.
- *Know What's for Lunch.* Get a weekly menu of school meals. Ask for nutrition facts so you can be sure the menu meets the Dietary Guidelines for Americans. Put it up on your refrigerator. Discuss all the healthy choices with your kids.
- *Team Up With the Food Service Staff.* Visit the school cafeteria. Get to know the staff. Let them know you value their services...and appreciate good daily nutrition for your child.
- *Plant a Seed.* Show your kids and their friends where healthy food comes from. Help your school start an edible landscape with a garden of goodies like fruits, vegetables, and herbs.
- *Throw a Tasting Party.* Volunteer to organize a classroom tasting party to introduce and encourage nutritious new foods the kids may never have tried.
- *Set Up a Group. Get involved.* Form a parent advisory committee for school meals. Recruit enthusiastic, "can-do" people to work with you.
- *Serve Your Kids Food for Thought.* Make sure kids appreciate how healthy breakfasts and lunches serve their minds as well as their bodies.
- *Listen.* If you listen to what your kids are learning at school about good nutrition, you can help them put their knowledge to work at home, too.

By being an active parent in your child's school, you're helping your children learn to enjoy good-tasting, good-for-them foods. By helping them develop good eating habits, you are improving their health.

Preparing Today's Children for a Healthier Tomorrow!

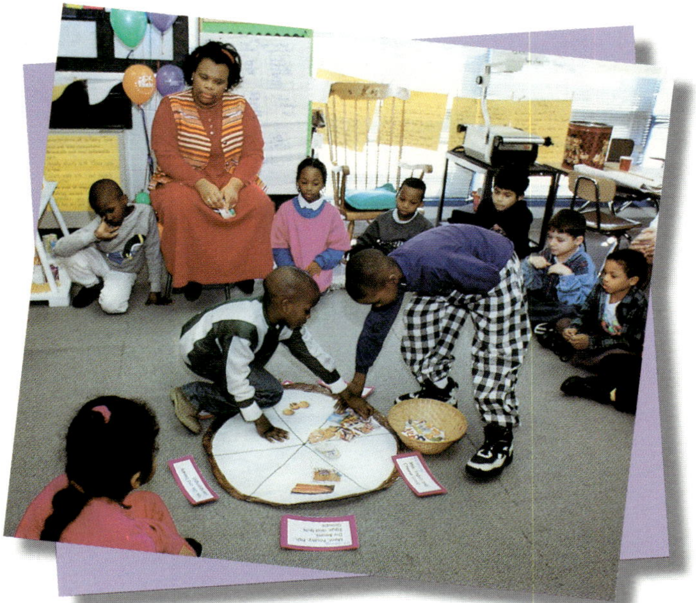

Secretary of Health and Human Services Donna E. Shalala says, "By developing good eating habits when we are young, we can help prevent health problems throughout our lives. Giving children the skills they need to improve their diets is a great investment in their long-term health and well-being."

Secretary of Education Richard W. Riley says, "Our first National Education Goal is that all children will start school ready to learn. We can all make sure that our children are ready to learn every day by reading with them at home and making sure that they have healthy meals. School breakfast and lunch programs are critical for states, communities and schools to reach this national goal. Any teacher can tell you that a hungry child cannot concentrate on the lesson and learn up to his or her ability."

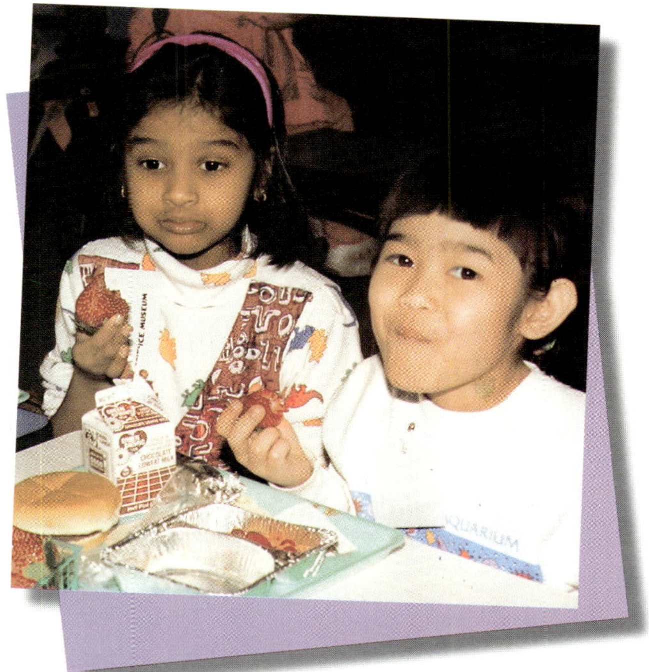

Notes